09

# The High-Risk Neonate: Part II

*Guest Editor*

M. TERESE VERKLAN, PhD, CCNS, RNC

# CRITICAL CARE NURSING CLINICS OF NORTH AMERICA

www.ccnursing.theclinics.com

*Consulting Editor*
JANET FOSTER, PhD, RN, CNS, CCRN

June 2009 • Volume 21 • Number 2



SAUNDERS an imprint of ELSEVIER, Inc.

**W.B. SAUNDERS COMPANY**
*A Division of Elsevier Inc.*

Elsevier Inc., 1600 John F. Kennedy Blvd., Suite 1800, Philadelphia, PA 19103-2899

http://www.theclinics.com

**CRITICAL CARE NURSING CLINICS OF NORTH AMERICA Volume 21, Number 2**
**June 2009 ISSN 0899-5885, ISBN-13: 978-1-4377-0465-5, ISBN-10: 1-4377-0465-4**

Editor: Katie Hartner
Developmental Editor: Donald Mumford



*Critical Care Nursing Clinics of North America* (ISSN 0899-5885) is published quarterly by Elsevier Inc., 360 Park Avenue South, New York, NY 10010-1710. Months of issue are March, June, September, and December. Business and Editorial Offices: 1600 John F. Kennedy Blvd., Suite 1800, Philadelphia, PA19103-2899. Periodicals postage paid at New York, NY and additional mailing offices. Subscription prices are $130.00 per year for US individuals, $233.00 per year for US institutions, $68.00 per year for US students and residents, $167.00 per year for Canadian individuals, $292.00 per year for Canadian institutions, $191.00 per year for international individuals, $292.00 per year for international institutions and $99.00 per year for Canadian and foreign students/residents. To receive student/resident rate, orders must be accompanied by name of affiliated institution, data of term, and the *signature* of program/residency coordinator on institution letterhead. Orders will be billed at individual rate until proof of status is received. Foreign air speed delivery is included in all *Clinics* subscription prices. All prices are subject to change without notice. **POSTMASTER:** Send address changes to *Critical Care Nursing Clinics of North America*, Elsevier Periodicals Customer Service, 11830 Westline Industrial Drive, St. Louis, MO 63146. **Customer Service: 1-800-654-2452 (US). From outside the United States, call 1-314-453-7041. Fax: 1-314-453-5170. E-mail: JournalsCustomerService-usa@elsevier.com (for print support) and JournalsOnlineSupport-usa@elsevier.com (for online support).**

*Reprints*. For copies of 100 or more of articles in this publication, please contact the Commercial Reprints Department, Elsevier Inc., 360 Park Avenue South, New York, New York, 10010-1710; Tel.: (212) 633-3813, Fax: (212) 462-1935, and E-mail: reprints@elsevier.com.

*Critical Care Nursing Clinics of North America* is covered in *MEDLINE/PubMed (Index Medicus), International Nursing Index, Nursing Citation Index, Cumulative Index to Nursing and Allied Health Literature, and RNdex Top 100.*

Printed in the United States of America.

# Contributors

## CONSULTING EDITOR

**JANET FOSTER, PhD, RN, CNS, CCRN**
Assistant Professor, College of Nursing, Texas Woman's University, Houston, Texas

## GUEST EDITOR

**M. TERESE VERKLAN, PhD, CCNS, RNC**
Associate Professor/Neonatal Clinical Nurse Specialist, University of Texas Health Science Center, School of Nursing, Houston, Texas

## AUTHORS

**DEBRA ARMENTROUT, RN, NNP, PhD**
Assistant Professor, Clinical Pediatrics, University of Texas Medical School, Houston, Texas

**DEBBIE FRASER ASKIN, MN, RNC**
Associate Professor, Faculty of Nursing; Faculty of Medicine, Department of Pediatrics, University of Manitoba; and Neonatal Nurse Practitioner, St Boniface General Hospital, Winnipeg, Manitoba, Canada

**CAROL CARRIER, MSN, RN, CNS**
Neonatal Clinical Nurse Specialist, Newborn Center, Texas Children's Hospital, Houston, Texas

**ANITA J. CATLIN, DNSc, FNP, FAAN**
Professor of Nursing and Ethics Consultant, Department of Nursing, Sonoma State University, Rohnert Park, California

**F. SESSIONS COLE, MD**
Park J. White, M.D., Professor of Pediatrics, Department of Pediatrics, Washington University School of Medicine; and Director, Chief Medical Officer, Division of Newborn Medicine, St. Louis Children's Hospital, St. Louis, Missouri

**WILLIAM DIEHL-JONES, RN, PhD**
Associate Professor, Faculty of Nursing; and Faculty of Science, Department of Biological Sciences, University of Manitoba, Winnipeg, Manitoba, Canada

**GEORGIA DITZENBERGER, NNP-BC, PhD**
Assistant Professor, Division of Neonatology, Department of Pediatrics, University of Wisconsin School of Medicine and Public Health; and Director, Neonatal Advanced Practice Nursing and Research, Meriter Hospital, Inc., Madison, Wisconsin

**JOAN RENAUD SMITH, MSN, RN, NNP-BC**
Neonatal Nurse Practitioner, Division of Nursing and Newborn Intensive Care, St. Louis Children's Hospital, St. Louis, Missouri

**LAURA STOKOWSKI, RN, MS**
Neonatal Intensive Care Unit, Inova Fairfax Hospital for Children, Falls Church, Virginia

**KAREN A. THOMAS, PhD**
Ellery and Kirby Cramer Professor, Department of Family and Child Nursing, University of Washington, Seattle, Washington

**M. TERESE VERKLAN, PhD, CCNS, RNC**
Associate Professor/Neonatal Clinical Nurse Specialist, University of Texas Health Science Center, School of Nursing, Houston, Texas

**DEBORAH VOLAT, BSN**
Registered Nurse, Oncology, John Muir Medical Center, Walnut Creek, California

**MARLENE WALDEN, PhD, APRN, NNP-BC, CCNS**
Professor of Clinical Nursing; and Director, Neonatal Nurse Practitioner & Acute Care Pediatric Nurse Practitioner Programs, School of Nursing, University of Texas, Austin, Texas

# Contents

**Preface** ix

M. Terese Verklan

**So, He's a Little Premature...What's the Big Deal?** 149

M. Terese Verklan

Health care providers have recently recognized that a large segment of the morbidity associated with preterm birth is disproportionately due to the late preterm infant (LPI). One explanation is that this population is the fastest-growing sector of all preterm births. This article describes the epidemiology and etiology of the LPI, and discusses why the LPI is at an increased risk for complications, such as thermal instability, hypoglycemia, feeding difficulties, respiratory distress, hyperbilirubinemia, and sepsis. The need for emergency department visits after hospital discharge and what is currently known regarding neurodevelopmental outcomes are also presented.

**Patient Safety: Effective Interdisciplinary Teamwork Through Simulation and Debriefing in the Neonatal ICU** 163

Joan Renaud Smith and F. Sessions Cole

According to the Institute of Medicine, team training is necessary to promote a safe and high-quality patient care environment. The complexity of the neonatal ICU requires that interdisciplinary teams collaborate, coordinate, and communicate to achieve common goals and support families. The use of strategies from the aerospace, nuclear power, and national defense industries—simulation, and debriefing—equips health care providers with the knowledge, skills, and behaviors necessary to perform effectively and safely. Families are encouraged to participate in simulation and debriefing so interdisciplinary teams can learn how to approach and support families when disclosing errors and to communicate sensitive information in a safe and nonthreatening environment.

**Nutritional Support of Very Low Birth Weight Newborns** 181

Georgia Ditzenberger

Nutritional support to promote optimal postnatal growth for very low birth weight (VLBW) newborns less than 1500 g at birth during the initial prolonged hospitalization is a significant issue. This article reviews the concepts involved in the nutritional support of VLBW newborns, including definitions and discussions of growth, optimal postnatal growth, body composition, initial weight loss, growth expectations, growth assessment tools used during the postnatal period, the relation between inadequate nutrition and neurodevelopment, the relation between protein intake and cognitive outcome, postnatal nutrition balance, the potential for programming of future adult-onset chronic conditions, a review of fetal nutritional intake, and current recommendations for nutritional support of VLBW newborns.

**Congenital Adrenal Hyperplasia: An Endocrine Disorder with Neonatal Onset** **195**

Laura Stokowski

Congenital adrenal hyperplasia (CAH) is a lifelong endocrine disorder that manifests acutely in the neonatal period. In the affected female newborn, CAH is associated with variable degrees of genital ambiguity that are extremely distressing to the new parents. The manner in which health care professionals react in the delivery room, newborn nursery, or neonatal intensive care unit in the early postnatal period is important. Insensitive or inappropriate statements cannot only be hurtful to families but are long remembered and can shape the attitude formed by parents toward their newborn.

**Retinopathy of Prematurity** **213**

Debbie Fraser Askin and William Diehl-Jones

This article briefly reviews the history of ROP followed by a discussion of the pathogenesis of this complex disorder. We describe the International Classification System for ROP and identify risk factors and screening recommendations. Finally, we discuss some of the measures that have been used in an attempt to both prevent and treat ROP.

**The Ten Commandments of Pain Assessment and Management in Preterm Neonates** **235**

Marlene Walden and Carol Carrier

Despite advances in pain assessment and management, nonpharmacologic and pharmacologic analgesic therapies continue to be underutilized in managing both acute and procedural pain in preterm neonates. Untreated acute, recurrent, or chronic pain related to disease or medical care may have significant and lifelong physiologic and psychological consequences. Painful procedures in the NICU may be unavoidable, so it is vital that caregivers balance the painful, medically necessary care with evidence-based nonpharmacologic and pharmacologic strategies to relieve pain and stress. We present Ten Commandments of pain assessment and management in preterm neonates to promote the use of best practices and compassionate care in the NICU.

**Living with Grief Following Removal of Infant Life Support: Parents' Perspectives** **253**

Debra Armentrout

Research findings reported in the literature about making life and death decisions for critically ill infants in the neonatal ICU focus primarily on the experiences of health care providers and the ethical dilemmas surrounding these decisions. Fewer studies focus on parents' experiences in making decisions about discontinuing life support for their infant, and even fewer address what life is like for parents following the deaths of their infants. This article expands on the concepts identified by parents as factors in their decision making and on the facilitators and barriers parents faced, and continue to face, in their grieving process.

**When the Fetus is Alive but the Mother is Not: Critical Care Somatic Support as an Accepted Model of Care in the Twenty-First Century?** **267**

Anita J. Catlin and Deborah Volat

There has been an increase in cases involving the maintenance of brain dead pregnant women on life support to allow for fetal growth toward viability and birth. This article provides an ethical analysis and discusses the critical care nursing needs of the maternal patient.

**When Neonatal ICU Infants Participate in Research: Special Protections for Special Subjects** **277**

Karen A. Thomas

Neonatal ICU research poses unique concerns for infants and parents. Children are considered a vulnerable research population. Federal regulations specify special protections when children participate in research. These regulations determine the types of research approvable for children based on the balance of risks and benefit. Risk also determines whether one or both parents' consent is required for their infant's participation in research.

**Index** **283**

## FORTHCOMING ISSUES

***September 2009***

**Neuroscience Nursing**
Anne W. Alexandrov, PhD, RN, CCRN, FAAN, *Guest Editor*

***December 2009***

**Obesity in Critically ill Patients**
Linda Harrington, PhD, RN, CNS, CPHQ, *Guest Editor*

## RECENT ISSUES

***March 2009***

**The High-Risk Neonate: Part I**
M. Terese Verklan, PhD, CCNS, RNC, *Guest Editor*

***December 2008***

**Innovative Practice Models for Acute and Critical Care**
Maria R. Shirey, PhDc, MS, MBA, RN, NEA-BC, FACHE, *Guest Editor*

***September 2008***

**Cardiovascular Disease in Women**
Lynn Smith Schnautz, RN, MSN, CCRN, CCNS, NP-C, *Guest Editor*

# Preface

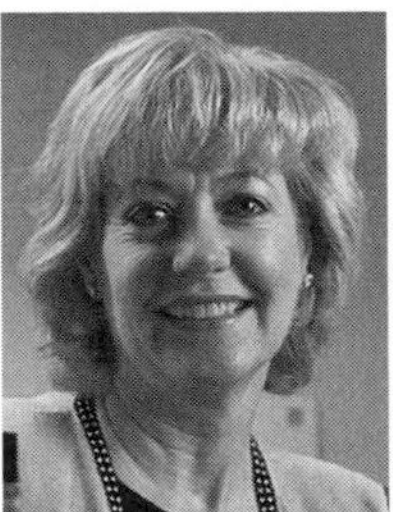

M. Terese Verklan, PhD, CCNS, RNC
*Guest Editor*

The past 10 years has witnessed dramatic changes in the care of all neonates, especially those requiring intensive care therapies. Our understanding of physiology, pathophysiology, diagnoses, and management has evolved such that mortality has decreased; however, increasing survival often means increasing morbidities. The youngest and the sickest of neonates do not always emerge from the neonatal ICUs unscathed. This issue is the second in a two-part series devoted to issues involving the high-risk neonate.

The re-emergence of kernicterus, an acute brain injury due to very high levels of bilirubin that results in permanent damage, caught many health care providers by surprise. This dreaded disorder was thought to be a thing of the past associated with severe Rh hemolytic disease. A closer look at who was developing hyperbilirubinemia and the reasons why has led to a closer inspection of how care is provided in the normal newborn setting. Until only a few years ago, any "healthy" baby born after 34 weeks' postmenstrual age was treated pretty much the same as a full-term baby. These "near-term" infants were expected to maintain their body temperature, take in sufficient enteral feeding, and be discharged within the customary 48 hours after birth. Early discharge did not provide a big enough window for health care providers to discover how much these babies were really struggling. An expert panel was convened to examine the issues, and it renamed the group of babies born between $34^{0/7}$ and $36^{6/7}$ weeks' menstrual age "late-preterm infants" to highlight their lack of maturity. The article "So He's a Little Premature: What's the Big Deal?" presents an overview of the most common problems that these newborns encounter in their first days of life.

I doubt that any health care provider today is unaware of the phrases "patient safety," "error reduction," "sentinel event," and "error disclosure." A change in the institutional culture from one of blame to one that invites discourse so that mistakes and harm are decreased is ongoing in many hospitals. Smith and Cole stress the importance of team communication and collaboration in "Patient Safety: Effective Interdisciplinary Teamwork Through Simulation and Debriefing in the Neonatal ICU." They discuss how ineffective communication can lead to a sentinel event and how

Crit Care Nurs Clin N Am 21 (2009) ix–xi
doi:10.1016/j.ccell.2009.04.001 

those patterns of communication may be modified. It has become clear that a toxic work environment is in large part responsible for medical errors, ineffective care, and promoting conflict and stress among the health care team. The creation of expert teams using simulation-based training and debriefing (eg, NeoSim) provides the opportunity for health care professionals to work together to improve teamwork skills (including communication) and to promote patient safety in real-life situations away from the bedside.

Traditionally, neonatal providers have been terrible in providing adequate nutritional support to the sickest neonate who is unable to tolerate enteral feeds. Although the use of percutaneous lines and improved hyperalimentation preparations have enhanced the nutritional status of neonates, many continue to be in a state of cachexia while in the neonatal ICU. In the article "Nutritional Support of Very Low Birth Weight Newborns," Ditzenberger discusses how inadequate nutrition may be responsible for postnatal growth restriction and a contributor to many of the chronic sequelae associated with very low birth weight infants. All neonates are expected to lose weight in the first days of life, much to their parent's disappointment, due to fluid shifts within the various compartments. Weight is a parameter that is tracked very closely and is key to medical management. A review of and recommendations for energy, fat, glucose, and protein intakes are presented. In addition, new research indicates that the neonatal ICU approach, which often encourages rapid growth of the tiny baby, may be laying the foundation for future adult onset of chronic disease such as central obesity and diabetes.

Stokowski discusses how advances in genetics and cell biology have positively impacted neonates born with endocrine dysfunction in "Congenital Adrenal Hyperplasia: An Endocrine Disorder with Neonatal Onset." It is uncomfortable for everyone in the delivery room when an excited mother wants to know, immediately after delivering her baby, whether it is a boy or a girl, and no one is able to give an answer because the genitalia are ambiguous. Stokowski reviews the endocrine system with respect to the adrenal hormones to better understand the pathophysiology, manifestation, and management of the neonate presenting with congenital adrenal hyperplasia. Sexual differentiation and other disorders of sexual development, along with the intricacies of gender assignment, are also presented. Strategies are reviewed to help families cope with these emotionally laden anomalies. A case study highlights the key points in the article.

Retinopathy of prematurity (ROP) has been recognized as a complication of prematurity for many years. There was a time when the disorder led to the development of blindness in huge numbers of babies due to their being placed in incubators with oxygen, whether they needed it or not. The epidemic of blindness scared neonatologists so much that many did not provide any oxygen to premature infants, causing increased mortality in some who would have likely lived. We continue to struggle today with trying to understand the pathophysiology of ROP and with weighing the risks and benefits of providing supplemental oxygen to immature babies. Askin and Diehl-Jones present the history of ROP and the classification system that is used to grade the disease. Risk factors and the development of ROP as we understand it are discussed. Recommendations for screening neonates and strategies to prevent the development of ROP and its progression are reviewed. Current interventions and investigational therapies are also discussed.

Any intensive care stay is fraught with multiple invasive procedures that seem to be repeated endlessly until discharge from the unit. The neonatal ICU is no different, although there has been a distinct trend to scrutinize whether each procedure is really needed. The pain response has been well studied in neonates, leaving no doubt that these very vulnerable patients experience a tremendous amount of pain. Research and clinical experience also detail that the more premature the infant, the less coping strategies the baby has in its arsenal; therefore, a preterm neonate is thought to be more sensitive than a full-term neonate. Walden uses a case study to illustrate the gaps that continue to remain between evidence-based practice and research findings. She uses a unique style, the "Ten Commandments," to drive home the message that all neonates need comprehensive pain assessment and management of that pain. Without evaluation of this fifth vital sign, health care providers are not practicing in an ethical manner or providing compassionate care.

I was fortunate to be invited to sit on a dissertation committee in which the doctoral candidate was examining how parents who made the decision to discontinue life support in the neonatal ICU felt about their decision years later. All members of the committee admitted that they could not read the results and discussion sections at the office because they were crying too much while reading what the parents said. Armentrout does a beautiful job of bringing the parent's perspective back to the neonatal health care provider in "Living with Grief Following Removal of Infant Life Support: Parents' Perspectives." The parents tell how they made their decision, the things they would have changed, and how they would like the neonatal team to better support them. She discusses the differences between the mother and the father in grieving, the parents' feelings of isolation, and how difficult it is when close friends and family do not recognize the parents' loss. The parents share how a shift in life priorities occurred as they began to move forward from the intense grief.

Catlin and Volat stimulate thought and ethical debate in "When the Fetus Is Alive but the Mother Is Not: Critical Care Somatic Support as an Accepted Model of Care in the Twenty-First Century?" Situations in which brain-dead women have been maintained on life support for the purpose of allowing the fetus to mature to viability have resulted in successful births in most cases. Ethical issues surrounding care of the mother, the special needs of the fetus, and the emotional needs of the involved family and the nurses delivering that care are examined through the use of insightful questions. The importance of teamwork among the obstetric and adult intensive care providers is also emphasized.

As a researcher who investigates physiologic instability in neonates requiring intensive care, I feel that the institutional review board process is often overly burdensome. I will admit, though, that it is a necessary evil, because there are some who do not always maintain integrity of the research process. Thomas provides a wonderful overview of the research process as it specifically relates to the neonate in "When Neonatal ICU Patients Participate in Research: Special Protections for Special Subjects." Neonates are a vulnerable population and cannot speak for themselves; thus, there must be a mechanism by which they have an advocate. Often, parents may not be able to seriously consider the ramifications of their baby being a research subject, given the emotions surrounding having a child in the neonatal ICU.

It has been a pleasure working with the article contributors for this issue and the past one. I sincerely thank the authors for taking the time to develop their work so that others may be stimulated by their thoughts.

M. Terese Verklan, PhD, CCNS, RNC
University of Texas Health Science Center
School of Nursing
6901 Bertner Avenue, Suite 565
Houston, TX 77459

E-mail address:
M.T.Verklan@uth.tmc.edu

# So, He's a Little Premature...What's the Big Deal?

M. Terese Verklan, PhD, CCNS, RNC

**KEYWORDS**

- LPI • Sepsis • Hyperbilirubinemia • Respiratory distress
- Hypoglycemia • Thermal instability • Feeding difficulties

Health care providers have recently recognized that a large segment of the morbidity associated with preterm birth is disproportionately due to the late preterm infant (LPI). One explanation is that this population is the fastest-growing sector of all preterm births. Originally these neonates were referred to as "near-term" infants. An expert panel convened to examine the growing issues surrounding this group of infants determined that the phrase did not capture how immature and vulnerable they are, however, and thus the term "late-preterm" infant was coined. The panel also came to consensus that the LPI is the neonate who is born between 34 weeks, 0 days, through 36 weeks, 6 days of gestation.[1] The 34th week was chosen because antenatal steroids to facilitate fetal lung maturation in the case of preterm labor would typically not be given.[2] This article describes the epidemiology and etiology of the LPI, and discusses why the LPI is at an increased risk for complications, such as thermal instability, hypoglycemia, feeding difficulties, respiratory distress, hyperbilirubinemia, and sepsis. The need for emergency department (ED) visits after hospital discharge and what is currently known regarding neurodevelopmental outcomes are also presented.

## EPIDEMIOLOGY OF THE LATE PRETERM INFANT

A preterm baby is one who is born before 37 weeks' postmenstrual age (PMA). The rate of preterm births is currently approximately 12.7%, an increase of more than 30% since the early 1980s (**Fig. 1**).[3,4] The LPIs are the fastest-growing subgroup of preterm babies and account for 75% of all preterm births (**Fig. 2**).[5] Concomitantly, there has been a decrease in the number of infants being delivered postterm, such that the most frequent length of a singleton pregnancy is now 39 weeks rather than 40 weeks of gestation.[3,5] Although non-Hispanic black neonates have preterm rates 1.5 times greater than Hispanic and non-Hispanic babies, the rate of non-Hispanic white LPIs increased the most overall, mainly because they account for the majority of births.[5] Interestingly, the mortality rate for the LPI is comparable to that for the

University of Texas Health Science Center, School of Nursing, 6901 Bertner Avenue, Suite 565, Houston, TX 77459
*E-mail address:* m.t.verklan@uth.tmc.edu

Crit Care Nurs Clin N Am 21 (2009) 149–161
doi:10.1016/j.ccell.2009.03.001 ccnursing.theclinics.com
0899-5885/09/$ – see front matter 

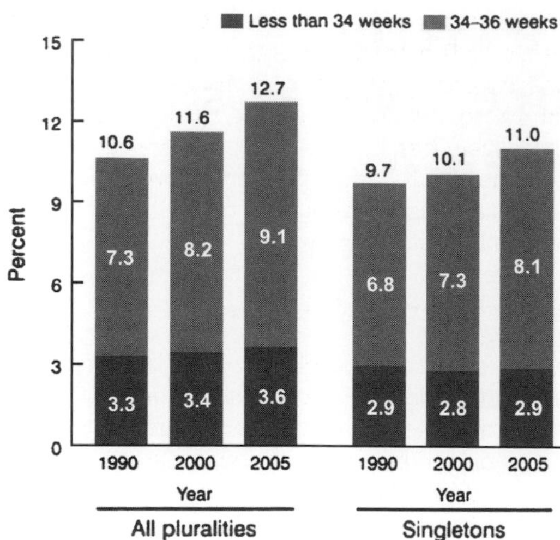


**Fig. 1.** Preterm birth rates in the United States for years 1990, 2000, and 2005. (*Data from* Martin JA, Hamilton BE, Sutton PD, et al. Births: final data for 2005. Natl Vital Stat Rep 2008;56:1–104.)

28- to 32-week PMA baby.[6] Studies have also shown that LPIs, when compared with term neonates, have an increased risk for mortality before their first birthday.[6,7]

## ETIOLOGY OF LATE PRETERM BIRTHS

Reasons the LPI birth rate has increased so dramatically over the last 10 years include increased maternal age, use of fertility treatments resulting in multiple gestations, and increasing obesity rates.[8] Preeclampsia, one of the most common medical complications of pregnancy, affects 5% to 10% of all pregnancies.[9] Delivery by induction or cesarean section is necessary if the mother or the fetus does not respond to medical management regardless of gestational age. It is a common obstetric practice to recommend delivery of the woman with preeclampsia at 34 weeks PMA.

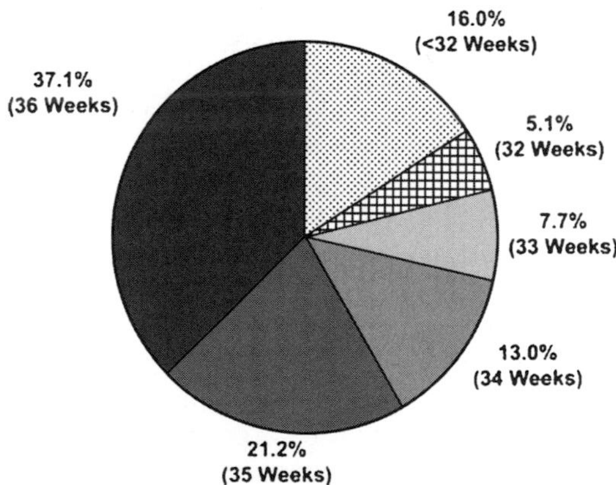


**Fig. 2.** Gestational age distribution of preterm births. (*Adapted from* Davidoff MJ, Dias T, Damus K, et al. Changes in the gestational age distribution among US singleton births: impact on rates of late-preterm birth, 1992 to 2002. Semin Perinatol 2006;30:9; with permission.)

Multiple gestation has had a significant effect on the LPI; the mean age at delivery for twins is 35.3 weeks.[10] The cesarean birth rate was at its highest ever at 29.1 in 2004.[11] Obstetricians increasingly performed cesarean sections on demand (parental request) at a rate of 4% to 18% of all cesarean deliveries.[10] In addition, the vaginal birth after cesarean delivery has been decreasing over the past decade. In general, there has been an increase in obstetric interventions in response to maternal preexisting conditions, such as diabetes.[12] Because of miscalculation of gestational age, there is a high risk for iatrogenic preterm delivery.

## COMPLICATIONS ASSOCIATED WITH LATE PRETERM INFANTS

From the health care provider's viewpoint, being born a few weeks early does not seem to place the neonate at risk. It is commonly believed that LPIs are "big" babies who can communicate their needs and therefore do not require special care or intensive care nursing. On closer inspection it becomes clearer that this population, although having different difficulties with transition to extrauterine life than the premature neonate less than 32 weeks PMA, certainly can be seen to be struggling with basic processes necessary for survival. Data indicate that there is a higher incidence of thermal instability, hypoglycemia, feeding difficulties, respiratory distress, hyperbilirubinemia, and sepsis than in the term population.

### *Thermal Instability*

One of the first physiologic issues neonatal healthcare providers learn is that even the healthy full-term neonate has a limited ability to maintain body temperature without assistance. The newly born infant leaves a warm, humid intrauterine environment and enters a delivery room that is cold and dry. Rapid heat loss by conduction and radiation occurs unless the neonate is placed into an environment that provides warmth and prevents heat loss, such as a prewarmed radiant warmer or, if the neonate is stable, placed directly onto the mother's chest and covered with a warm blanket. Preterm babies are even more predisposed to cold stress because they have a larger surface area in relation to their body mass, limited brown fat stores, and decreased subcutaneous fat. Less muscle tone or activity increases their body surface area that is exposed to the environment. The more preterm the neonate, the more immature the epidermal barrier is, which results in an increased transepidermal water loss.[13] Ideally, all neonates should be in a neutral thermal environment, which is a physiologic state in which the infant maintains a normal temperature without increasing oxygen consumption, burning glucose or brown fat stores for nonshivering thermogenesis.[14]

Immediately after delivery the infant is dried and covered in warmed blankets. Axillary temperatures should be monitored every 30 minutes to 1 hour during the transitional period.[14,15] Rectal temperatures are no longer the standard of care because the risk for rectal perforation and vagal stimulation is high.[13] A decrease in the axillary temperature alerts the nurse to intervene early to prevent failure of the body's heat-regulation mechanism and a resultant decrease in the core temperature.[14] The first bath should be delayed until the body temperature has stabilized at 36.3 to 36.9°C (97.3–98.6°F).[14] The temperature should be taken at least 30 minutes after the bath and 1 hour after transfer to an open bassinet, assessing the temperature every 4 hours until stable. Unless signs of temperature instability appear, the temperature should be obtained every 8 hours until discharge.[14]

Symptoms of cold stress include apnea, bradycardia, lethargy, hypotonia, poor feeding, pallor and mottled appearance. Metabolic acidosis, increased metabolic rate, and pulmonary vasoconstriction may also occur.[13] LPIs can significantly increase oxygen consumption when they are not maintained within a neutral thermal environment.[16] A cold neonate will not be warmed by simply swaddling him in warm blankets. Immediately the nurse should place the neonate on a prewarmed radiant warmer or skin-to-skin on the mother's chest. The nurse should also investigate the cause of the hypothermia by determining how the heat was lost, through mechanisms of conduction, radiation, convection, or evaporation. For example, there may have been many visitors and the baby was unswaddled for a prolonged period in a cool room. In that scenario, heat may have been lost by conduction to the cool bed surface, by convection because of cold air currents, and by radiation of the baby's body heat to the cooler surfaces in the room. During rewarming, the neonate needs to be closely observed to detect apnea, tachycardia, or overheating if the body temperature increases too quickly (>0.5°C or 0.9°F).

Before discharge, the nurse must be confident that the neonate is able to maintain his or her temperature while in the bassinet and dressed with appropriate clothing. Parents need to be aware of symptoms of temperature instability, such as changes in breathing, color, and feeding behaviors. They should be taught how to correctly obtain an axillary temperature and to call the pediatrician for temperatures that exceed the normal ranges. Cold stress is one of the more common reasons for parents to take their child to the ED.[17] The parents should verbalize understanding of how to properly bath the baby using techniques that minimize heat loss. It should be emphasized that they should dress their baby in layers as they are dressed to suit the environmental temperatures and assist the baby in maintaining body temperature.[18]

### *Respiratory Distress*

LPIs have an increased incidence of respiratory distress (28.9%) as compared with the full-term neonate (4.2%),[19] making it the most common complication for this age group.[20] PMA of 34 weeks, 0 days, through 36 weeks, 6 days marks the end of the terminal sac period of lung development.[21] The alveolar saccules are maturing into alveoli lined with type I epithelial cells that are being brought into close proximity with capillary loops to facilitate gas exchange. Type II cells, responsible for the secretion of surfactant and maintenance of low surface tension within the alveoli, begin to cluster at the alveolar ducts and proliferate as the lung surface area rapidly begins to increase.[21,22] Concomitantly, the synchrony and control of breathing is beginning to emerge, such that by term, the risk for apnea of prematurity should be minimal.[22]

Respiratory distress is an acute disorder presenting within an hour or two after birth and accompanied by signs of increased work of breathing, such as increasing tachypnea, flaring, retractions, and grunting.[23] Given the immaturity of the lung structure and function of the LPI, there may be delayed absorption of fetal lung fluid and surfactant insufficiency, both of which contribute to decreased pulmonary compliance and increased pulmonary resistance. A trial of labor and a vaginal delivery results in the release of catecholamines that circulate in the neonate in the hours after delivery. The catecholamines, especially epinephrine, facilitate the absorption of lung fluid and the release of surfactant, such that pulmonary compliance continues to improve over the hours following delivery. Many LPIs are delivered by cesarean section without a trial of labor, however, which places them at high risk for developing transient tachypnea of the newborn, respiratory distress syndrome, pulmonary hypertension, and hypoxic respiratory failure.[8,24] de Almeida and colleagues[25] found that one in every seven LPIs required more resuscitation procedures during transition to extrauterine life when delivered by elective cesarean section.

The neonatal nurse is responsible for assessing the neonate's work of breathing immediately on delivery to determine the need for pulmonary support, such as oxygen supplementation or positive pressure ventilation. Within 2 hours of birth a complete physical examination of all body systems should be performed to evaluate the risks for developing complications that may interfere with a successful adaptation to extrauterine life.[14,15] A respiratory assessment includes vital sign determination, rate, depth and pattern of respirations, and evaluation of work of breathing and air entry. A persistent pattern of tachypnea needs to be investigated because this is the first sign that the body is requiring increased delivery of oxygen to the alveoli. Nasal flaring, grunting, and retractions often subside over the first hours of life as fetal lung fluid is absorbed by the lymphatic system. Because LPIs often present with a delay in respiratory transition, it is recommended that respiratory status be evaluated at least once every 4 hours during the first 24 hours of life, and then once per shift until discharge unless otherwise warranted.[15,23,24]

When symptoms of respiratory distress are evident the nurse should notify the nurse practitioner/physician and request evaluation the LPI's clinical condition. The nurse should place a pulse oximeter probe to evaluate oxygenation, and if appropriate provide a heated, humidified supplementation oxygen source.[21,23] A diagnosis of respiratory distress typically means the baby will need intravascular access for the provision of fluids and electrolytes, including glucose and often calcium. The nurse must rule out or manage common causes of respiratory distress, such as thermal instability, hypoglycemia, and feeding difficulties.

### *Hypoglycemia*

At birth, blood glucose levels are estimated to be 70% to 80% of maternal levels.[14,26] To maintain euglycemia, hepatic glycogenolysis and gluconeogenesis must be initiated. Before delivery, there is an increase in plasma catecholamines, a surge in glucagon concentrations, and a decrease in circulating insulin.[14,26] There is an impressive increase in fat oxidation and available amino acids are also converted to glucose. Serum glucose levels in all babies fall to the lowest nadir between approximately 1 and 2 hours of life. The postnatal decrease in glucose concentrations is greater in the preterm than the full-term neonate, however. Compensatory mechanisms should then stabilize the glucose levels between 40 and 100 mg/dL within 2 to 4 hours, even if the neonate is not fed soon after birth. Hepatic glycogen is rapidly consumed if early feeds or a glucose source are not initiated. The neonate then depends on gluconeogenesis and lipolysis to maintain a normal glucose level. It is estimated that 8% of neonates develop hypoglycemia in the first 4 hours of life.[27] The incidence of hypoglycemia in the preterm infant is approximately three times that of the term neonate, with 66% requiring intravenous dextrose support.[26]

There are several reasons that the LPI is at high risk for developing hypoglycemia. First, preterm infants have decreased glycogen and adipose stores as a result of being born early. The immature hepatic enzyme systems for gluconeogenesis limit their ability to increase glucose production in response to increased metabolic demands. Glucose-regulated insulin secretion by the pancreas is also immature, such that there may be high levels of circulating insulin despite decreased levels of serum glucose.[26] LPIs commonly have medical complications, such as respiratory distress syndrome, hypothermia, sepsis, perinatal stress/hypoxia, and decreased oral intake, that require increased substrate availability. Inadequate glucose supply/production is the most common cause of neonatal hypoglycemia. The neonate typically requires 4 to 6 mg/kg/min, much greater than that required by an adult.[26,27]

The definition of what constitutes hypoglycemia is controversial, and is believed to be on a continuum in which the individual neonate and clinical circumstances need to be taken into consideration. Hypoglycemia is commonly diagnosed when the plasma glucose level decreases to less than 40 to 45 mg/dL, although many believe the cutoff level should be increased to 55 to 70 mg/dL.[26,27] Signs and symptoms are variable, making the diagnosis of hypoglycemia difficult if the health care provider is not vigilant. Nurses should make frequent, regular assessments to detect nonspecific symptoms or be suspicious, given the neonate's clinical condition, when there are no obvious symptoms present (**Box 1**).

The brain uses approximately 80% of the total glucose that is available.[26] Two major glucose transporter isoforms carry glucose to the neurons and the astrocytes. GLUT1 is predominately located in the blood–brain barrier and in astrocytes (glia), and GLUT2 is found in neurons. Astrocytes also store glycogen, which may be an immediate source of glucose in times of physiologic stress. Other substrates, such as ketones and lactate, are actively transported to the astrocyte by the monocarboxylate transporter (MCT) 1 and into neurons by MCT2.[26,27] When glucose levels decrease, lactate can then be used as an alternate energy source. The "lactate shuttle" is an important protective mechanism because LPIs are not capable of mounting an adequate counterregulatory ketogenic response to hypoglycemia. In contrast to the term neonate, the LPI is not able to effectively use other alternative fuels, such amino acids, free fatty acids, ketone bodies, and glycerol.[28] Because of immature protective mechanisms in the brain, the LPI is at risk for neurologic sequelae if hypoglycemia is not detected and treated in a timely fashion.

Monitoring for hypoglycemia begins before the infant's birth. The perinatal/neonatal nurse should be aware of any preexisting maternal conditions or adverse events that occurred during labor and delivery that may increase the risk for hypoglycemia.

**Box 1**
**Signs and symptoms of hypoglycemia**

*Cardiopulmonary changes*

Apnea

Bradycardia or tachycardia

Tachypnea

Grunting

Respiratory distress

Color changes (pallor, cyanosis, mottling)

*Neurologic changes*

Irritability, excessive crying, high-pitched or weak cry

Lethargy, stupor

Hypotonia, limp,

Jitteriness, tremors

Seizures

Changes in the level of consciousness

*Other*

Hypothermia

Poor feeding

*Data from* Refs.[14,16,26,27]

Maternal conditions may include diabetes, preterm labor and use of tocolytics, or hypertensive disorders of pregnancy. Intrapartum events may include fetal bradycardia, chorioamnionitis, abruptio placenta, and perinatal asphyxia/hypoxia requiring resuscitative interventions.

Within 30 to 60 minutes of age, a screening plasma glucose test should be obtained in the LPI who is demonstrating symptoms of hypoglycemia or is at high risk for developing hypoglycemia.[14] A glucose value less than 40 mg/dL warrants investigation and intervention.[14] The enzymatic reagent strips used for point-of-care testing have well-known shortcomings. They may underestimate the true glucose level and are sensitive to user errors.[27] They do function satisfactorily as a screening tool, however, with serum specimens sent for laboratory confirmation to establish the diagnosis. Hypoglycemia is a medical emergency, and as such, intervention should not wait until the laboratory has determined the serum glucose value.

Prevention or correction of hypoglycemia may be done by providing early, frequent enteral feedings in the stable LPI. Breastfeeding should be initiated in the delivery room and occur at 2- to 3-hour intervals, whereas the formula-fed infant should be fed every 3 to 4 hours.[14,29] A repeat screening plasma glucose test should be repeated 30 to 60 minutes after the feeding, along with reevaluation of the neonate's clinical condition. If the hypoglycemic infant is refusing or not tolerating the feedings, an order should be obtained to provide an intravenous bolus of 2 mL/kg of D10W to be given "push" followed immediately with an infusion of D10W at 4 to 6 mg/kg/min or 80 mL/kg/day.[14,27,30] Serial blood glucose screening should be performed at 4-hour intervals, or sooner depending on the degree of hypoglycemia, the response to glucose/feedings, presentation of symptoms, and trends over time, until the risk period has passed.[14,27,30] Parent teaching is also a nursing priority in that the parents need to be aware of the symptoms of hypoglycemia and the importance of frequent feedings to maintain euglycemia and establish successful breastfeeding/formula feeding.

### *Feeding Difficulties*

Establishing enteral feeding is often problematic for both maternal and neonatal reasons. The mothers may experience delayed lactogenesis, in which the milk comes in after day 3, because of factors that contributed to the premature delivery itself.[31,32] LPIs may experience difficulty with latch and coordination of the breathe-suck-swallow reflex. Their effectiveness of milk removal and stimulation of the breast in the first days of breastfeeding may not be adequate,[31] which may also contribute to slow milk production. In addition, obesity, diabetes, hypertensive disorders of pregnancy, and cesarean section, common reasons for preterm birth, have been associated with decreased levels of prolactin in the mother in response to suckling.[32–36] Prolactin is important in the production of early milk as opposed to continuing lactation.[32]

LPIs are commonly cared for in the postpartum setting, as one part of the healthy mother–infant dyad. The postpartum nurse or neonatal nurse may be largely unaware of the factors that may negatively affect successful lactation and enteral feeding. Compared with the term baby, the LPI tends to be sleepier, has a less vigorous suck, and tires more easily. It is known that preterm infants have immature sucking patterns whether feeding from the bottle or the breast.[37,38] Cues signaling hunger are often not well developed. These characteristics may be interpreted by the health care provider as early signs of sepsis and result in the neonate being separated from the mother for a septic work-up and observation, often leading to an interruption in breastfeeding.

Difficulties with feeding easily translate into increased risks for hypoglycemia, cold stress, dehydration, hyperbilirubinemia, and weight loss; therefore, the nurse must monitor the baby's physiologic stability during feeds. Feeding issues are the most common cause for increased length of stay.[39] Poor feeding and hypoglycemia required intravenous fluid in 27% of LPIs as compared with 5% of term infants.[39,40] The mother and the health care team need to be patient, creative, and flexible in assisting the baby to feed successfully. The LPI may need to be awakened to feed 8 to 12 times in a 24-hour period. Because the infant may not completely empty the breast, the mother should be instructed on ways to express the milk to promote optimal milk production.[31]

It has been recommended that nurses observe breastfeeding every 3 hours, and that the baby be weighed before and after breastfeeding to confirm adequate breast milk intake.[41,42] It is also recommended that a lactation consultant observe the mother–baby dyad breastfeeding on a daily basis; the consultant can be helpful with suggestions, such as use of nipple shields to facilitate the baby's latch and suck and to stimulate milk production. Before hospital discharge, there should be documentation that the neonate has been successfully bottle or breastfeeding for at least 24 hours.[18] The mother must also be aware that feeding issues may appear after discharge and that the pediatrician should be notified as soon as possible to prevent complications and rehospitalization.[18]

### *Hyperbilirubinemia*

Hyperbilirubinemia, or jaundice, is the most common cause of hospitalization in the first week of life for all neonates.[43] All infants become jaundiced because of an imbalance between bilirubin production and elimination. Neonates have a shorter erythrocyte life, increased erythrocyte volume, and immature physiologic pathways necessary for conjugation of bilirubin. In addition, the LPI who has feeding difficulties often has decreased gastrointestinal motility with subsequent reuptake of conjugated bilirubin that further contributes to the increased bilirubin load on the hepatocyte.[18,43] The LPI who is exclusively breastfeeding has a high risk for developing severe hyperbilirubinemia that if left untreated may progress to kernicterus.[43,44] Kernicterus is an acute bilirubin encephalopathy that results in permanent brain damage, hearing loss, dentition problems, and cerebral palsy. Almost every infant reported to the U.S. Pilot Kernicterus Registry, most of whom are LPIs, were noted to have suboptimal breastfeeding as the predominant cause for this debilitating disease.[43,44]

The practice of treating LPIs as term neonates with typical hospital discharge at 48 hours after delivery is in part responsible for the increase in severe hyperbilirubinemia noted in EDs. LPIs are almost twice as likely to develop severe hyperbilirubinemia compared with term infants, and more importantly, the peak in bilirubin increase in the LPI does not occur until days 5 to 7 of life, several days after hospital discharge.[45] Any baby that presents with jaundice in the first 24 hours of life is considered to have pathologic hyperbilirubinemia that must be investigated.[46]

The nurse is responsible for evaluating feeding patterns and enteral intake, especially in the LPI who is breastfeeding.[47] Because visual assessment of jaundice is not always accurate, bilirubin screening using serum total or transcutaneous bilirubin is recommended. There are standing orders that permit the nurse to obtain a serum total bilirubin (STB) if the nurse notes jaundice or increased levels of transcutaneous bilirubin. The STB value should be plotted on the hour-specific bilirubin nomogram to assist in the prediction of the LPI's risk for developing severe hyperbilirubinemia that will require intervention.[44–47] The nurse is also responsible for providing the parents with verbal and written information regarding how to recognize symptoms of hyperbilirubinemia and the importance of notifying their healthcare provider when this occurs. A follow-up appointment with the pediatrician should be made within 72 hours of hospital discharge. The nurse should document in the baby's record that the mother was given the date and time of the follow-up appointment and that she verbalized understanding of the discharge education and the importance of keeping the follow-up visit with the pediatrician.

### *Sepsis*

Every preterm baby can be thought of as being immunocompromised because of the immaturity of the immune system. Indeed, one of the causes of preterm labor and preterm birth is maternal chorioamnionitis, along with the risk that the newly born infant may acquire an infection during delivery. Early-onset sepsis presents within the first 72 hours and is almost always caused by perinatally acquired infections.[48,49] The most common pathogens are group B streptococci and *Escherichia coli*.[48,49] In addition to chorioamnionitis, risk factors for developing sepsis include preterm premature rupture of membranes for greater than 18 hours, maternal fever, and preterm delivery.[48,49] LPIs are at more risk than term neonates because they are born before term, the time when maternal antibodies are completely transferred to the fetus.[16,48]

Health care providers need to have a high degree of suspicion regarding sepsis, because it is one of the most difficult disorders to diagnose.[48,49] Failure to recognize early-onset sepsis contributes to morbidity, mortality, and increased length of stay. The conundrum is that the presenting symptoms of sepsis are the same as other disorders common to preterm infants. Temperature instability, respiratory distress, change in feeding patterns, hypoglycemia, lethargy, irritability, and hyperbilirubinemia are some of the most common signs of sepsis. The nurse must be aware of the LPI's increased susceptibility for sepsis and be cognizant of maternal risk factors that may place the neonate at risk. The nurse should also recognize those neonatal risk factors that predispose the LPI to sepsis, such as perinatal asphyxia, difficult delivery, male gender, black race, and multiple gestation.[48] Because these infants have decreased maternally acquired passive immunity, adherence to infection control practices, including hand washing, is essential.

## EMERGENCY DEPARTMENT VISITS

Before hospital discharge the mother is given an appointment for a follow-up visit with a primary pediatric care provider. In addition to evaluating the LPI soon after discharge, the appointment gives the mother entrée to community resources that she can access if she has concerns regarding her baby. LPIs use EDs and are readmitted to the hospital more often than full-term infants.[17,18,20] It has been found that 4.3% of LPIs as compared with 2.7% term infants who were discharged early (less than two-night hospital stay) had a period of observation in the ED or were readmitted.[50] A total of 77.1% of LPIs and 60.3% of term infants had an admission diagnosis of hyperbilirubinemia and sepsis.[50] An interesting finding from the same study was that non-breastfed LPIs and term infants had no difference in hospital readmission; however, breastfed LPIs were 2.2 times more likely to be readmitted than breastfed term infants.[50]

The age of the infant at hospital presentation varied according to weeks of prematurity. Full-term babies were taken to the ED more commonly during the second week of life, whereas most LPIs presented during the fourth week of life.[17] Of these LPIs, the overwhelming proportion consisted of 36-week PMA infants.[17] One explanation for the finding is that the 34- and 35-week PMA infants may have had a longer stay in the hospital, whereas the 36-week infant was viewed as a healthy neonate and discharged as if it was a term baby.[17]

LPIs and term infants delivered by cesarean section presented to the ED more than those neonates who were delivered vaginally.[3,17] It may be that the increase in cesarean section rates and elective deliveries are contributing to an increase in iatrogenic prematurity.[3] Six diagnoses accounted for approximately 75% of all diagnoses of both LPIs and full-term infants, and were the same for all neonates: gastrointestinal disorders, respiratory distress, fever, hyperbilirubinemia, sepsis, and feeding problems.[17] Almost 37% of LPIs who presented to the ED within the first month of life required readmission and had an average length of stay of 5.7 days.[17] Although there is limited evidence that documents the LPI's hospital course after the initial nursery discharge, it is clear that this cohort of neonates contributes significantly to increased costs of health care.

## NEURODEVELOPMENTAL OUTCOME

Just as data are being collected regarding the increased health care costs associated with the LPI population, researchers are beginning to document the impact of being born 4 to 6 weeks premature on neurodevelopmental outcome. It is known that a significant amount of brain development has yet to occur during this time. The cortical volume of the brain of a 34-week PMA infant is only 50% of that of the full-term neonate, highlighting the tremendous amount of brain growth, development, and neural networking that remains to be completed.[51] The LPI is extremely vulnerable to any injury that may increase the risk for neural injury or disruption in neuronal and glial development during this critical period of growth.[51]

Severe intraventricular hemorrhage (IVH) and periventricular leukomalacia (PVL) are major neurodevelopmental complications common to the preterm neonate, with the risks decreasing with increasing gestational age. Although IVH traditionally has not been thought of in association with the LPI, the germinal matrix is not fully involuted until 36 weeks PMA.[51] The germinal matrix, the most common site for hemorrhage, is also the place from which cerebral and glial precursor cells originate. Injury to the site may negatively affect neuronal development.[51] The LPI is not routinely screened for IVH or its sequelae during the initial hospitalization or on follow-up visits to a primary pediatric health care provider.

The LPI is also not routinely screened for PVL, a well-known predictor of adverse neurodevelopmental outcome. Because 50% of the brain is undergoing rapid growth, development, and organization, the LPI is at high risk for white matter damage.[51] Chorioamnionitis and early-onset sepsis are also associated with white matter injury and negative neurologic outcomes.[28,52] Researchers have documented changes in the microstructural development of central white matter and its descending fibers in infants who have white matter injury.[51,53] Although studied in infants younger than 34 weeks PMA, it has been found that perinatal white matter injury is associated with a decreased volume of gray matter and myelinated white matter when reaching 40 weeks' gestation.[54]

Early data suggest that LPIs will significantly affect the education system and the costs of providing education. Within the first 3 years of life, LPIs had a higher incidence of being diagnosed with developmental delay and were referred for special needs preschool resources more frequently than term infants.[54] LPIs also were found to have increased difficulties with school readiness. An improved understanding of neurologic injury in the LPI and how neurodevelopmental outcomes are negatively affected is necessary before optimal neuroprotective strategies can be developed.

## SUMMARY

The LPI has only recently become recognized as a population with increased morbidity and mortality, and so a paucity of information remains. Because they constitute such a large proportion of preterm births, even a small increase in their birth rate will have a considerable impact on short- and long-term health care and educational and productivity costs. It has been estimated that $51,600 is associated with the birth of each preterm infant.[18] What makes a neonate high risk needs to take into account the full clinical picture rather than an arbitrary birth weight of 1500 g or less. Morbidity and mortality from respiratory distress, sepsis, feeding issues, hyperbilirubinemia, and hypoglycemia continue to be substantial. Despite recommendations from the American Academy of Pediatrics[17] and the Association of Women's Health, Obstetric, and Neonatal Nurses,[42] the LPI continues to be discharged early. Health care providers need to reconsider how care for the LPI is approached from both a medical and a nursing perspective, and hospital policies and clinical guidelines must be changed to specifically address the needs of this distinctive population.

## REFERENCES


1. Raju TNK, Higgins RD, Stark AR, et al. Optimizing care and outcome for late-preterm (near-term) infants: a summary of the workshop sponsored by the National Institute of Child Health and Human Development. Pediatrics 2006; 118:1207–14.
2. Cunningham FG, Leveno KJ, Bloom SL, et al. Williams obstetrics. 22nd edition. New York: McGraw-Hill; 2005.
3. Davidoff MJ, Dias T, Damus K, et al. Changes in the gestational age distribution among US singleton births: impact on rates of late-preterm birth, 1992 to 2002. Semin Perinatol 2006;30:8–15.
4. Martin JA, Hamilton BE, Sutton PD, et al. Births: final data for 2005. Natl Vital Stat Rep 2008;56:1–104.
5. Raju TNK. Epidemiology of late preterm (near-term) births. Clin Perinatol 2006;33: 751–63.
6. Kramer MS, Demissie K, Yang H, et al. The contribution of mild and moderate preterm birth to infant mortality. JAMA 2000;284:843–9.
7. Joseph KS, Kramer MS, Allen AC, et al. Gestational age- and birthweight-specific declines in infant mortality in Canada, 1985–94. Paediatr Perinat Epidemiol 2000; 14:332–9.
8. Shaw RR. Late preterm birth: a new nursing issue. MCN Am J Matern Child Nurs 2008;33:287–93.
9. Sibai BM. Hypertension. In: Gabbe G, Niebyl JR, Simpson JL, editors. Obstetrics: normal and problem pregnancies. 5th edition. Philadelphia: Churchill Livingstone; 2007. p. 863–912.
10. Lee YM, Cleary-Golmand J, D'Alton ME. The impact of multiple gestations on late preterm (near-term) births. Clin Perinatol 2006;33:777–92.
11. March of Dimes. Preterm birth overview. Available at: http://marchofdimes.com/peristats/tlanding.aspx?reg=99&lev=0&top=3&slev=1&dv=qf. Accessed January 23, 2009.
12. Shapiro-Mendoza CK, Tomashek KM, Kotelchuck M, et al. Effect of late-preterm birth and maternal medical conditions on newborn morbidity risk. Pediatrics 2008;121:e223–32.

13. Brand MC, Boyd H. Thermoregulation. In: Verklan MT, Walden M, editors. Core curriculum for neonatal intensive care nursing. 4th edition. St. Louis (MO): Elsevier; 2009. p. 110–9.
14. Verklan MT. Adaptation to extrauterine life. In: Verklan MT, Walden M, editors. Core curriculum for neonatal intensive care nursing. 4th edition. St. Louis (MO): Elsevier; 2009. p. 72–90.
15. American Academy of Pediatrics and American College of Obstetricians and Gynecologists. Guidelines for perinatal care. Washington, DC: AAP/ACOG; 2007.
16. Blackburn ST. Maternal, fetal and neonatal physiology. A clinical perspective. 3rd edition. St. Louis (MO): Saunders Elsevier; 2007.
17. Jain S, Cheng J. Emergency department visits and rehospitalizations in late preterm infants. Clin Perinatol 2006;33:935–45.
18. Engle A, Tomashek KM, Wallman C, et al. "Late-preterm" infants: a population at risk. Pediatrics 2007;120:1390–401.
19. Wang ML, Dorer DJ, Fleming MO, et al. Clinical outcomes of near-term infants. Pediatrics 2004;114:372–6.
20. Escobar GJ, Clark RH, Greene JD. Short term outcomes of infants born at 35 and 36 weeks gestation: we need to ask more questions. Semin Perinatol 2006;30: 28–33.
21. Askin DF. Respiratory distress. In: Verklan MT, Walden M, editors. Core curriculum for neonatal intensive care nursing. 4th edition. St. Louis (MO): Elsevier; 2009. p. 453–83.
22. Hansen TN, Corbet A. Control of breathing. In: Taeusch HW, Ballard RA, Gleason CA, editors. Avery's diseases of the newborn. 8th edition. Philadelphia: Saunders; 2005. p. 616–33.
23. Whitsett JA, Rice WR, Warner BB, et al. Acute respiratory disorders. In: MacDonald MG, Mullett MD, Seshia MMK, editors. Avery's neonatology: Pathophysiology and management of the newborn. 5th edition. Philadelphia: Lippincott; 2005. p. 553–77.
24. Dudell GG, Jain L. Hypoxic respiratory failure in the late preterm infant. Clin Perinatol 2006;33:803–30.
25. de Almeida MFB, Guinsburg R, da Costa JO, et al. Resuscitative procedures at birth in late preterm infants. J Perinatol 2007;27:761–5.
26. Garg M, Devaskar SU. Glucose metabolism in the late preterm infant. Clin Perinatol 2006;33:853–70.
27. Armentrout D. Glucose management. In: Verklan MT, Walden M, editors. Core curriculum for neonatal intensive care nursing. 4th edition. St. Louis (MO): Elsevier; 2009. p. 172–81.
28. Volpe JJ. Neurology of the newborn. 5th edition. Philadelphia: Saunders; 2008.
29. American Academy of Pediatrics. Section on breastfeeding. Breastfeeding and use of human milk. Pediatrics 2005;115:496–506.
30. McGowan JE, Price-Douglas W, Hay WW Jr. Glucose homeostasis. In: Merenstein GB, Gardner SL, editors. Handbook of neonatal intensive care. 3rd edition. St. Louis (MO): Mosby; 2006. p. 368–90.
31. Meier PP, Furman LM, Degenhardt M. Increased lactation risk for late preterm infants and mothers: evidence and management strategies to protect breastfeeding. J Midwifery Womens Health 2007;52:579–87.
32. Walker M. Breastfeeding the late preterm infant. JOGN Nurs 2008;37:692–701.
33. Chapman DJ, Perez-Escamilla R. Maternal perception of the onset of lactation is a valid, public health indicator of lactogenesis stage II. J Nutr 1999;130: 2972–80.

34. Chapman DJ, Perez-Escamilla R. Identification of risk factors for delayed onset of lactation. J Am Diet Assoc 1999;99:450–4.
35. Rasmussen KM, Kjolhede CL. Prepregnant overweight and obesity diminish the prolactin response to suckling in the first week postpartum. Pediatrics 2004;113: e465–71.
36. Nissen E, Uvnas-Mobergb K, Svenssonc K, et al. Different patterns of oxytocin, prolactin but not cortisol release during breastfeeding in women delivered by caesarean section or by the vaginal route. Early Hum Dev 1996;45:103–18.
37. Medoff-Cooper B, Verklan MT, Carlson S. Nutritive sucking and physiological correlates in very low birthweight infants. Nurse Res 1993;42:100–5.
38. Medoff-Cooper B, Bilker W, Kaplan J. Sucking behavior as a function of gestational age: a cross-sectional study. Infant Behav Dev 2001;24:83–94.
39. Adamkin DH. Feeding problems in the late preterm infant. Clin Perinatol 2006;33: 831–7.
40. Ip S, Chung M, Kulig J, et al. An evidence-based review of important issues concerning neonatal hyperbilirubinemia. Pediatrics 2004;114:e130–53.
41. Stellwalgen L, Boies E. Care of the well newborn. Pediatrics 2006;27:89–97.
42. Askin DF, Bakewell-Sachs S, Medoff-Cooper B, et al. Late preterm infant assessment guide. Washington, DC: Association of Women's Health, Obstetric and Neonatal Nursing; 2007.
43. Watchko JF. Hyperbilirubinemia and bilirubin toxicity in the late preterm infant. Clin Perinatol 2006;33:839–52.
44. Bhutani VK, Johnson L. Kernicterus in late preterm infants cared for as term healthy infants. Semin Perinatol 2006;30:89–97.
45. Sarici SU, SErdar MA, Korkmaz A, et al. Incidence, course and prediction of hyperbilirubinemia in near-term and term newborns. Pediatrics 2004;113:775–80.
46. American Academy of Pediatrics Subcommittee on Hyperbilirubinemia. Management of hyperbilirubinemia in the newborn infant 35 or more weeks of gestation. Pediatrics 2004;114:297–316.
47. Bradshaw WT, Watson RL. Gastrointestinal disorders. In: Verklan MT, Walden M, editors. Core curriculum for neonatal intensive care nursing. 4th edition. St. Louis (MO): Elsevier; 2009. p. 589–637.
48. Lott JW. Immunology and infectious disease. In: Verklan MT, Walden M, editors. Core curriculum for neonatal intensive care nursing. 4th edition. St. Louis (MO): Elsevier; 2009. p. 694–723.
49. Benjamin DK, Stoll BJ. Infection in late preterm infants. Clin Perinatol 2006;33: 871–82.
50. Tomashek KM, Shapiro-Mendoza CK, Weiss J, et al. Early discharge among late preterm and term newborns and risk of neonatal mortality. Semin Perinatol 2006; 30:61–8.
51. Adams-Chapman I. Neurodevelopmental outcome of the late preterm infant. Clin Perinatol 2006;33:947–64.
52. Adams-Chapman I, Stoll B. Neonatal infection and long term neurodevelopmental outcome in the preterm. Curr Opin Infect Dis 2006;19:290–7.
53. Huppi PS, Murphy B, Maier SE, et al. Microstructural brain development after perinatal cerebral white matter injury assessed by diffusion tensor magnetic resonance imaging. Pediatrics 2001;107:455–60.
54. Inder TE, Huppi PS, Warfield S, et al. Periventricular white matter injury in the premature infant is followed by reduced cerebral cortical gray matter volume at term. Ann Neurol 1999;46:755–60.

# Patient Safety: Effective Interdisciplinary Teamwork Through Simulation and Debriefing in the Neonatal ICU

Joan Renaud Smith, MSN, RN, NNP-BC[a,*], F. Sessions Cole, MD[b,c]

**KEYWORDS**

- Team communication and collaboration
- Error disclosure • Crew resource management (CRM)
- SBAR • Family-centered care • Simulation

A decade has passed since the Institute of Medicine's (IOM's) report concluded that up to 98,000 lives are lost annually in United States hospitals as a result of error, and national efforts to improve health care safety have become a priority.[1] Patient safety has been defined by the IOM as the "prevention of harm to patients;"[2] this prevention of harm includes "freedom from accidental or preventable injuries produced by medical care."[3] Patient safety is indistinguishable from quality health care and is the foundation of care delivery.[2] Health care errors and poor quality of care are the products of a complex health care system faced with increased costs, rapid advances in information and technology, and the lack of quality and quantity of clinical evidence needed to guide clinical decision making.[4] Because of the complexity of most health care organizations, many health care errors are related to the systems and processes within these organizations. Many health care errors are preventable and have resulted in both death and an economic consequence as high as $29 billion dollars annually.[1] The complexity and dynamics of most neonatal ICUs (NICUs) place medically fragile

[a] Division of Nursing and Newborn Intensive Care, St. Louis Children's Hospital, One Children's Place, St. Louis, MO 63110, USA
[b] Department of Pediatrics, Washington University School of Medicine, 660 S. Euclid Avenue, St. Louis, MO 63110, USA
[c] Division of Newborn Medicine, St. Louis Children's Hospital, One Children's Place, St. Louis, MO 63110, USA
* Corresponding author.
*E-mail address:* joanrs@bjc.org (J.R. Smith).

Crit Care Nurs Clin N Am 21 (2009) 163–179
doi:10.1016/j.ccell.2009.01.006 ccnursing.theclinics.com
0899-5885/09/$ – see front matter 

infants at high risk for encountering errors during their stay. These infants are defenseless compared with physiologically more mature newborns, older children, and adults and leave little margin for error. It is the responsibility of health care organizations and neonatal care providers to ensure the safety of these vulnerable infants. Although some errors occur at the point of service (eg, a nurse administering the wrong medication), most errors result from flaws within the health care system or facility design (eg, excessive noise levels or miscommunication).[5] High-reliability organizations that foster a culture of safety promote evidence-based practice, focus on system improvements, and provide favorable working conditions to nurses, physicians, and other care providers dedicated to high-quality and safe care.[6]

To deliver high-quality patient care, a culture of safety should start with the vision and direction of hospital leaders. Senior leaders are instrumental in promoting and establishing a culture of safety and should engage important front-line staff (eg, nurses, physicians, therapists, pharmacists, support staff) at the ground level to form interdisciplinary teams to identify and mitigate patient harm. Mitigating harm is best accomplished by designing reliable health care processes and developing an appropriate culture of safety.[7] Nurses play a key role in promoting patient safety. According to the IOM, there is a strong link between nursing, patient safety, and quality of care.[2] Nurses are at the core of intercepting errors and preventing harm to patients and are responsible for coordinating and integrating multiple aspects of quality within the context of patient care delivery; therefore nurses must assume a leadership role in optimizing high-quality and safe care.[8] The Agency for Health care Research and Quality and the Robert Wood Johnson Foundation jointly have developed a handbook for nurses on patient safety and quality. *Patient Safety and Quality: An Evidence-Based Handbook for Nurses* highlights the evidence surrounding a broad range of issues involved in providing high-quality and safe care across various health care settings.[6] Error reduction is possible as nurses and all members of the health care team become more aware of their roles in patient safety and are able to implement evidence-based safety and improvement strategies. Situational awareness and the knowledge and skills associated with safety must become routine nursing practice.

## COMMUNICATION FAILURE AND SENTINEL EVENTS

It is the responsibility of all members of the interdisciplinary health care team, both as team members and as individual practitioners, to assure they are delivering safe, high-quality care. Effective communication among all team members is an essential component for the safe delivery of care. Ineffective communication or the lack of communication among team members promotes an environment in which medical errors can occur. More than two thirds of the sentinel events reported to the Joint Commission[9] (formerly known as the Joint Commission on Accreditation of Healthcare Organizations) were caused primarily by failures in communication. Communication failures were the leading root cause of sentinel events from 1995 to 2004. In 2008, the Joint Commission issued a Sentinel Event Alert titled *Behaviors that Undermine a Culture of Safety,* stating that disruptive and intimidating behaviors threaten the performance of the health care team, jeopardizing the quality and safety of patients, and that health care organizations must address these problem behaviors to promote a culture of safety.[9] Health care organizations need to offer tools to promote positive teamwork, collaboration, and effective communication.

Historically, health care organizations have tolerated unprofessional and disruptive behaviors. Often disruptive behaviors are not reported because of fear of retaliation and the possible stigma associated with "blowing the whistle" on a colleague or because of an overall reluctance to confront the intimidator.[9] In fact, according to a survey on intimidation by the Institute for Safe Medication Practices[10] of more than 2000 health care providers from hospitals (N = 1565 nurses, 354 pharmacists, 176 others), 40% of clinicians have remained silent or passive during patient care events rather than question a known intimidator. Nearly half (49%) of all respondents reported that previous experiences with intimidation had altered the way they handle order clarifications or questions about medication orders, and three quarters (75%) had asked colleagues to help them interpret an order or validate its safety so that they did not have to interact with an intimidating prescriber. Unfortunately, only 60% of respondents believed their organization had clearly defined effective processes in place to handle disagreements about the safety of an order, and only 39% believed that their organization dealt effectively with intimidating behavior. These negative behaviors coupled with poor communication can lead to mistrust, chronic stress, and dissatisfaction among nurses, resulting in nurses leaving their positions and profession.[11] Unhealthy work environments contribute to medical errors, ineffective care, and conflict and stress among health professionals. In 2005, the American Association of Critical-Care Nurses published national standards for establishing and sustaining healthy work environments[11] that complement and support the American Nurses Association[12] and the IOM recommendations.[13–15] The Joint Commission issued a new Leadership Standard addressing disruptive and inappropriate behavior effective January 1, 2009. Accrediting institutions must have a code of conduct defining acceptable, disruptive, and inappropriate behaviors and a process for managing these inappropriate behaviors with an emphasis on zero tolerance.[9]

## INTERDISCIPLINARY TEAMS: RESPECT, COLLABORATION, AND COMMUNICATION

Because of the complexity of most NICUs, neonatal health care professionals caring for extremely vulnerable infants often work in highly stressful and emotionally charged environments that can contribute to intimidating and disruptive behavior, especially when coupled with fatigue.[9] The combination of complexity, a hierarchical authority structure, poor communication, and a culture deeply rooted in individual professional autonomy creates barriers to establishing a safe culture.[16] According to the IOM's report, *To Err is Human: Building a Safer Health System*,[1] health care providers rarely are trained as teams but instead tend to be trained as individuals, even though they function almost exclusively as teams. More errors in the delivery of health care are caused by poorly performing systems than by individual performance. Therefore, the IOM recommends interdisciplinary team training to enhance patient safety and the quality of health care.[1] As neonatology has become increasingly complex, the need for interdisciplinary teams to collaborate and coordinate their care to achieve a common goal (improved patient outcomes) and to support patients/families is essential. The IOM's report, *Health Professions Education: A Bridge to Quality*, states "patients and families commonly report that caregivers appear not to coordinate their work or even to know what each other is doing [p. 31]."[15] Defining teams and team-related terms is important for clarity (**Box 1**). A team is a small number of people who have complementary skills, whose work is interdependent, and whose members are committed to a common purpose, performance goals, and approach for which they are mutually accountable.[17] "Teamwork" refers to behaviors that facilitate effective interaction among team members.[18] "Interdisciplinary teams" refers to a partnership between or among two or more health professionals/disciplines who collaborate to achieve shared decision making according to patient-centered goals and values and optimization of the composite team's knowledge, skills, and perspectives, with mutual respect and trust

**Box 1**
**Definition of terms**

Adverse event: an untoward, undesirable, and usually unanticipated event, such as death of a patient, an employee, or a visitor in a health care organization[75]

Collaboration: the interaction between health care professionals that enables the knowledge and skills of both professionals synergistically to influence the delivery of patient care[23]

Crew resource management: a communication methodology used to train flight crews in critical communication and decision making, stress management, and team building which can be an effective strategy in enhancing teamwork and lowering risks[44,45]

Debriefing: facilitated discussions designed to assist learners in the reflection process regarding the learning experience, used as a tool to close the gap between the experience and making sense of the experience[60,70]

Error: An act of commission (doing something wrong) or omission (failing to do the right thing) that leads to an undesirable outcome or to significant potential for such an outcome[3]

Error disclosure: "communication between a health care provider and a patient, family member, or patient proxy that acknowledges the occurrence of an error, discusses what happened, and describes the link between the error and outcomes in a manner that is meaningful to the patient/family [p. 760]"[32]

Handoff: the transfer of important or necessary information and the responsibility for care of the patient from one health care provider to another[76]

Interdisciplinary team: a partnership between two or more health professionals/disciplines who collaborate to achieve shared decision making according to patient-centered goals and values and to optimize the composite team's knowledge, skills, perspectives, and mutual respect and trust among all team members[19]

Multidisciplinary team: health care professionals from several disciplines working side-by-side but independently from one another[20]

Near miss: an event or situation that did not produce patient injury but only because of chance. This good fortune might reflect robustness of the patient (eg, a patient who has penicillin allergy receives penicillin but has no reaction) or a fortuitous, timely intervention (eg, a nurse happens to realize that a physician wrote an order in the wrong chart).[3]

Patient safety: the prevention of harm to patients,[2] including freedom from accidental or preventable injuries produced by medical care[3]

Respect: the act of "esteeming another, an act that demands we ourselves have a sense of authenticity, integrity and self-knowledge [p. 149]"[22]

Safety culture: a commitment to safety that permeates all levels of an organization, from frontline personnel to executive management[3]

SBAR (situation, background, assessment, and recommendation): a communication tool to standardize discussion and information sharing among caregivers to ensure that patient information is delivered consistently and accurately, especially during critical events, shift handoffs, or patient transfers[62]

Sentinel event: an unexpected occurrence that causes significant physical or psychological harm or death or has the risk of causing significant harm. Serious injury specifically includes loss of limb or function. Such events are called "sentinel" because they signal the need for immediate investigation and response.[75] Sentinel event alerts are published for organizations accredited by the Joint Commission and interested health care providers. These alerts identify specific sentinel events, describe their common underlying causes, and suggest steps to prevent occurrences in the future. These alerts can be accessed at: http://www.jointcommission.org/SentinelEvents/SentinelEventAlert/.[75]

Simulation: re-creation of an actual event that has occurred previously or could potentially occur [p. 306][47]

Transparency: a process in which errors are fully disclosed to patients/families.[38]

among all team members.[19] Unlike interdisciplinary teams, multidisciplinary teams incorporate health care professionals from several disciplines working side-by-side but independently. The difference between interdisciplinary and multidisciplinary teams lies in the interaction among team members.[20] Effective interdisciplinary teams require members to develop trust for one another's judgments and expertise.

Mutual respect, trust, confidentiality, responsiveness, empathy, effective listening, and communication among all clinical team members are necessary for promoting teamwork and shared decision making.[21] Teams require strong organizational support to function effectively. Health care organizations need to have processes in place to support and foster interdisciplinary teamwork and collaboration. Respect is an ethical principle, the cornerstone for all critical care relationships, and is the first step toward establishing a healthy relational environment among health care professionals and families. Many definitions of "respect" exist. Essentially, it is the act of "esteeming another, an act that demands we ourselves have a sense of authenticity, integrity and self-knowledge [p. 149]."[22] When health care professionals respect one another and individual family members by honoring each other's choices, preferences, and boundaries for privacy, regardless of their beliefs or uniqueness, a sense of acceptance and worthiness is experienced, resulting in a healthy health care work environment.[22] Collaboration is the interaction between health care professionals that enables the knowledge and skills of both professionals to influence the delivery of patient care synergistically.[23] Collaboration includes team members' sharing knowledge with a joint effort in the intellectual planning of work, nonhierarchical team decision making, and readiness to assume responsibility for patient outcomes.[24,25] Communication and collaboration among team members are vital to creating and sustaining a culture of safety.

Mutual participation is key to establishing an interdisciplinary collaborative relationship. No one discipline provides patient care in isolation; therefore, health care professionals should collaborate with one another by assuming complementary roles, working together cooperatively, and sharing responsibility for problem solving and decision making. Physicians and nurses should collaborate and increase team members' awareness of each others' knowledge and skills, leading to an improvement in decision making. Interdisciplinary teams need to approach decision making and plans of care as a joint effort undertaken on behalf of the patient with a common goal from all disciplines.[20] Communication among team members must flow freely regardless of the authority gradient. Clinical decision making should be shared among all members of the health care team. Improved team collaboration and communication have been described by health care professionals as being among the most important factors in improving clinical effectiveness and job satisfaction.[26] High-performance teams do not happen by chance. Building effective teams requires more than assembling a group of individuals together in one place; it requires planning, training, practice, and leadership. Teams need to be taught specific behaviors to function effectively, and health care organizations need to provide team members with support for and access to education that develops critical communication skills including self-awareness, inquiry/dialogue, conflict management, negotiation, advocacy and listening.[11]

An effective team involves commitment, competence, communication, coordination and agreement on common goals for the patient.[17] Expanding on the definition, the five "C's" include

1. Common goal: Every team member shares the short- and long-term goals of the team/organization. The common goal for clinical teams is patient centered and outcomes directed.

2. Commitment: Every team member is committed to attaining the goals that have been mutually set.
3. Competence: Every team member has the knowledge, skills, behaviors, and attitudes necessary to perform his or her role.
4. Communication: Team members communicate effectively/efficiently with each other, the patient, and other groups or individuals.
5. Coordination: Team members work together efficiently and effectively.

When all five "C's" are present, clearly defined, and uninhibited by intimidation, patient outcomes can be improved, and the risk of patient harm can be reduced.

## COMMUNICATION AND FAMILIES

Effective communication among health care professionals is important in preventing errors and promoting quality of care, but the need for effective communication does not stop at the health care team itself. Families of critical care patients are concerned about the adequacy, reliability, and timeliness of communication.[27,28] Shared decision making requires health care professionals to provide effective and consistent communication, coupled with respect, to families. Patient and family needs and preferences should be central to care delivery in the NICU, and everyone's point of view should be heard and considered in a respectful environment.[22] The IOM identified six aims for the redesign of health care[14] and called on health care organizations to provide care that is safe, effective, patient-centered, timely, efficient, and equitable, urging hospitals to put patients first. Patient-centered care is pivotal in the prevention of medical errors.[1] Families are at the core of delivering patient-centered care in the NICU, and family-centered care is vital to promoting patient safety. Families should be encouraged and empowered to act as partners and collaborators with the health care team in shared decision making. Improving quality and safety by bringing families into the planning, delivery, and evaluation of health care is the foundation of family-centered care.[29] The policy statements in the American Academy of Pediatrics' *Family-Centered Care and the Pediatrician's Role*[30] provide a summary of the core principles of family-centered care and include specific recommendations on how to integrate family-centered care in hospitals, clinics, and the community. Research suggests that when health care providers and administrators partner with patients and families, the quality and safety of health care rise, costs decrease, and provider and patient satisfaction increases.[29]

### *Error Disclosure*

Partnering with and communicating effectively with families are important in the daily delivery of care but are especially important when any treatments or procedures result in patient outcomes that differ significantly from anticipated outcomes.[31] "Error disclosure" refers to "communication between a health care provider and a patient, family member, or patient proxy that acknowledges the occurrence of an error, discusses what happened, and describes the link between the error and outcomes in a manner that is meaningful to the patient/family [p. 760]."[32] Patients desire error disclosure—transparency—and practitioners agree that errors causing harm should be disclosed, but a significant gap exists between patients' desires and clinical practice.[33–37] This process can be challenging for health care providers. Most patients/families wish to be informed of adverse events. Prompt, compassionate, and honest communication with patients and families following an incident is essential, and restoring trust is critical.[38] How the communication process is handled strongly influences the reactions of patients and their families. Health care professionals need to take responsibility and apologize when an error occurs. The apology helps restore the patient's dignity and begin the healing process, and it also helps health care providers deal with their own emotional trauma.[38] Failing to admit the error and not openly expressing regret can add insult to injury by not fully respecting the patient/family's situation.

Although most health care providers generally support error disclosure, there are barriers that inhibit them from talking to patients: difficulty in acknowledging their mistakes, fear of litigation, intense shame or guilt, or the lack of training in making a disclosure.[34] Health care professionals hold themselves to very high standards and therefore may find it difficult to deal with failure. Because of the emotional effects of these events on both the patient/family and caregiver, communication failures often are the reason a patient or family files a malpractice suit. A wide variation exists in disclosing errors. Because of the lack of standards and training, health care providers may have difficulty delivering bad news.[39] Health care professionals need to know how to support both families and their colleagues when errors are disclosed. Error disclosure is a behavioral skill that traditionally is not taught in nursing or medical school, but it can be taught to members of the health care team in a safe and nonthreatening environment.

### *Caregiver Support after Error Disclosure*

Debriefing and support of caregivers following an adverse event is extremely important. Like patients and families, caregivers are affected emotionally and functionally by an adverse event and frequently are an unrecognized "second victim." Training is needed in supporting colleagues when they are the "second victim."[40] Interdisciplinary teams are in position to support one another. Organizations need to offer health care professionals assistance in managing the stress of the adverse event so healing can occur and the member(s) can return to work comfortably and take better care of patients.[40] Health care providers, risk managers, and other support personnel need training in communicating with patients and colleagues and should be taught how to debrief as a team after an adverse event.[38,40]

Coaching health care team members in ways to provide information to the family in a direct and honest manner during the emotionally intense period immediately after an incident can be critical for maintaining a compassionate and trusting relationship. Simulation training, including training in behavioral skills in communicating adverse events, in coaching others in this skill, and in providing support after experiencing an adverse event, should be provided for nurses, physicians, and other clinicians, as well as department chairs and managers.[38]

## BARRIERS TO EFFECTIVE COMMUNICATION AND TEAMWORK

Unfortunately, effective communication and teamwork do not always exist in real clinical settings. Their absence may be the result of low expectations within a system's culture.[20] Adverse clinical events and outcomes have been related to social, relational, and organizational structures that have contributed to communication failures.[41] Poor communication and ineffective collaboration and teamwork result in disruptive behaviors and can affect negatively staff relationships, staff satisfaction and turnover, and patient outcomes.[20,42,43]

Barriers to communication and collaboration can occur within disciplines but frequently occur across disciplines. Nurses and physicians interact several times during a shift, but often each individual has a different perception of his or her own role and different responsibilities toward the patient that can lead to their having different goals.[20] Multiple barriers to effective communication and collaboration exist. A specific barrier that dramatically compounds nurse–physician collaboration, communication, and teamwork is cultural differences. Because clinicians in the United States come from a variety of countries and cultural backgrounds, cultural differences can exacerbate communication problems.[31] Gender influences and hierarchical models of authority also have been identified as barriers to communication and teamwork.[20] Hierarchical models position physicians at the top, resulting imbalances in knowledge and power and a potentially false sense of team collaboration and communication although nurses and other staff perceive communication failures. When hierarchies exist, people on the lower end tend to refrain from speaking up or attending to a specific problem. Individuals at the top of the hierarchy can present themselves as intimidating and unapproachable, hindering communication and placing patients in harm's way.[31] Organizational support and interdisciplinary leadership and teamwork are essential in establishing a zero-tolerance policy for abusive and intimidating behavior among all members of the health care team.

## EFFECTIVE METHODS FOR ENHANCING INTERDISCIPLINARY TEAMWORK AND COMMUNICATION

It can be challenging to assemble teams in the NICU that work together long enough to achieve effectiveness over time. Often, depending on the discipline, clinical responsibilities rotate among attending staff, bedside staffing is restricted because of shortages, and medical residents spend limited time in the NICU. Because patient comorbidities in the NICU are extremely complex, and human factor performance may limit clinicians' recognition of rapidly evolving problems, it is crucial for clinicians to have standardized communication tools and environments that proactively support effective communication. Health care has turned to other complex, high-risk industries for strategies to reduce errors and accident rates and to improve teamwork. In aviation, crew resource management (CRM) is a communication methodology used to train flight crews in critical communication and decision making, stress management, and team building that can be an effective strategy in enhancing teamwork and lowering risks.[44,45] Structured communication tools with standardized language and procedures that replace hierarchical relationships with mutual decision making have been adopted from the aviation industry to assist practitioners in daily decision making.[44] The goal of CRM is to organize members of a team to think and act as a team with the common goal of safety.[46] CRM teaches team communication and highlights errors in a simulated setting in the hope of avoiding the same error in a real-life setting involving humans. It teaches that all members of a team are vital and that if a team member at any level believes that something is not being done appropriately or in the best interest of the team or other people who have put their trust in the team, then that member must speak up.[47] Health care professionals need to recognize their own limitations, cognitive errors, and stressors such as fatigue that can degrade their performance and contribute to errors and mistakes.[44] Recognizing these limitations and eliminating certain behaviors to reduce errors are part of the CRM training.

Using CRM, individual team members are trained for specific roles and can fill this role on any team to which they are assigned. This approach allows each individual to function in his or her assigned role on multiple teams and allows members of the team to come and go without effecting team function. For example, using CRM training techniques, when a code is called in the NICU, each team member takes a position at the infant's bedside that communicates his or her training and abilities to other members of the team. Each individual member has a clear role; there is no confusion, and a leader always is identified who is decisive and encourages all members to participate.

The CRM strategies of team training, simulation, interactive group debriefings, and measurement of crew performance have been shown to improve the operation of flight crews and the safety of air travel significantly. These same strategies have been applied widely[48] in neonatal care,[49–51] in emergency departments,[52,53] in pediatric ICUs,[53] and in operating rooms.[54–56] Despite the interest and research, no studies have shown that CRM training can improve teamwork and quality of care.[57,58] Therefore, it is hoped that improved teamwork and communication will improve patient outcomes and safety, but more research is needed.

## HANDOFFS

Today's health care system has become more specialized, with greater numbers of health care providers involved in patient care, resulting in more fragmentation across multiple settings. An essential component of health care communication is communicating the critical information needed to transfer the responsibility for a patient's care from one health care provider to another. According to the IOM, safety often fails first because of inadequate handoffs.[14] Too often, effective communication is situation or personality dependent.[59] The process of handoff is complex, involving communication about patients at shift changes and between care providers, and requires a mechanism for accurately, efficiently, effectively transferring information within complex organizational systems.[60] The Joint Commission requires that all health care providers implement a standardized approach for handoff communication, including an opportunity to ask and respond to questions.[61]

## SITUATION, BACKGROUND, ASSESSMENT, AND RECOMMENDATION

The situation, background, assessment, and recommendation (SBAR) technique is a shared model for standardized communication designed to facilitate and improve interdisciplinary communication. Communication styles vary among physicians and nurses, each discipline having its own terminology and idiosyncrasies, partly because of training. Physicians are instructed to be very concise and to focus on bullets of critical information; nurses are trained to be more descriptive of clinical situations.[59] This standardized communication tool has been shown to be effective in bridging the difference in communication styles.[62] The SBAR technique is an easy-to-remember tool used to improve handoffs, especially critical conversations, by providing a framework for communication between members of the health care team about a patient's condition.[20] The NICU often is chaotic and hurried; critical information can fall through the cracks at handoffs, and communication also can be misunderstood. For example, a potential for error can occur when verbal orders for medication are written down by someone other than the prescriber and then are transcribed onto an order form by a third person. Used extensively in medicine, and originating from the nuclear submarine service, SBAR is a communication tool to standardize discussion and information sharing among caregivers to ensure that patient information is delivered consistently and accurately, especially during critical events, shift handoffs, or patient transfers.[62] The SBAR technique meets the Joint Commission's National Patient Safety Goals,[61] requiring organizations to implement a standardized approach to handoff communications. SBAR provides a shared mental model for all clinicians to use during handoffs or transfers (**Box 2**).

**Box 2**
**Example of SBAR communication**

Situation: What is happening at the present time? *Baby boy Johnson is having persistent apneic spells.*

Background: What are the circumstances leading up to this situation? *Earlier in my shift, I added a blanket to maintain Baby Johnson's temperature and noted he had emesis following two of his enteral feedings. He also has a central line from his abdominal surgery 2 weeks ago.*

Assessment: What do I think the problem is? *I don't think he looks right, and I'm afraid he may be septic.*

Recommendation: What should we do to correct the problem? *I need you to come in immediately and assess the patient. He may need a sepsis evaluation, antibiotics started, and, if he continues to be apneic, he may need positive pressure ventilation.*

## STRATEGIES TO TEACH INTERDISCIPLINARY TEAMWORK AND COMMUNICATION

### *Simulation*

Simulation-based training is growing in recognition as an instructional strategy incorporating adult learning theory, real-time clinical situations, and video debriefing to allow teams an opportunity to improve their knowledge, to practice skills, and to gain expertise while evaluating their performance.[63] Simulation also can help capture the complexity of teamwork in a real-world setting and provide opportunities for health care professionals to grow and learn together, focusing on the creation of expert teams instead of expert individuals.[64,65] The IOM suggests the use of simulation exercises to enhance teamwork as one of the mechanisms for improving patient safety.[1] "Simulation refers to the recreation of an actual event that has previously occurred or could potentially occur [p. 306]"[47] and can provides learners an opportunity to experience real-life scenarios and interventions in clinical situations within a safe, controlled, supervised setting without posing risks to patients.[66] Simulation exercises can occur off units in a laboratory or in situ (meaning in the original place). In situ simulation provides training in the setting where patient care is delivered and real errors occur.[65] During in situ simulation training, a health care team is asked to care for a simulated patient (a mannequin or an actor) during a critical medical event. The entire simulation is videotaped. This type of real-life training is standard operating procedure in commercial aviation, aerospace, nuclear power, and the military and now is being applied in health care settings.[67,68]

Simulation can take many forms including relatively simple or complex strategies. Human patient simulators are among the most recent technological advances used as an instructional method in medical and nursing education. Interactive mannequins, or realistic human-patient simulators, are programmed to provide realistic physiologic responses such as respirations, pulses, and heart and breath sounds. Advanced models can communicate with the learner, responding to real-time questions during the simulation exercise, and can provide learners with the opportunity to develop and maintain clinical competencies.[66] The success of simulation programs is based on carefully designed clinical scenarios that are aligned with the needs of the learner and on skillfully led debriefings.[69] Simulation can provide a replication of the neonatal environment, equipped with the technology and the models of equipment that will be encountered in the NICU, as well as complex scenarios that require successful team interactions. Technical or procedural, cognitive, and behavioral skills can be simulated also, allowing for teamwork and competency checks. Leadership skills during emergent situations can be enhanced throughout the use of role simulation by improving communication skills as they relate to discussions about futility of medical care or end-of-life decision making.

Neonatal resuscitation is a high-risk and uncommon event. Health care providers caring for newborns may have limited opportunities to participate in extensive resuscitation efforts and to maintain their competency. Providing neonatal practitioners the opportunity to participate in simulation-based resuscitation training allows them to maintain competency in a safe and controlled environment. Through the use of simulation, team-training methods have been incorporated into the neonatal resuscitation program to provide teams the opportunity to rehearse team components as well as to learn technical skills and build trust.[49] Launched in 1997, NeoSim was the first neonatal simulation-based training program located at Packard Children's Hospital on the campus of Stanford University.[70] NeoSim is a successful, innovative training program designed to develop skills and maintain competency for neonatal resuscitation[51,71] The success of this program is based on its methodology, not on complex or expensive technology. Most of the trainees who participated in the NeoSim program reported that their learning occurred during the follow-up facilitated debriefing sessions.[69]

### *Debriefing*

Debriefings occur immediately after a simulated scenario and are led by experienced instructors. Although simulation provides specific clinical scenarios, it is the debriefing that allows health care team members to evaluate their own performance and system processes. Debriefings are facilitated discussions designed to assist learners in the reflection process regarding the learning experience and are used as a tool to close the gap between the experience and making sense of the experience[63,72] Using video-recorded simulation scenarios, an experienced instructor poses open-ended questions during the debriefing to help learners through the evaluation process. The goal of this questioning process is to incorporate the process of reflection as a tool that enables the learners to grow.[63] Together the learners can view concrete examples of technical (assembling and inserting the chest tube), cognitive (knowledge of a disease process or the indications for a chest tube), and behavioral skills (communication, leadership, and teamwork). Learners are able to reflect as individuals and as a team. As a team, learners can begin to piece together why a specific situation was successful or what they could have done differently in a real-life emergency.

Simulation provides a forum that enables individuals to learn as members of an interdisciplinary team and provides a safe environment for Individual members to discuss and share their experience as they uncover system failures and collectively solve problems. Experiential learning during simulation becomes effective when the focus is directed towards the human factors necessary for team performance rather than technical skills. The learner's personal experience and insight during the debriefings teach other participants about communication and teamwork in a structured and safe environment in which sensitive issues and difficult team situations can be addressed without shame, guilt, and embarrassment that may occur when reviewing a real-time adverse event.[65] Information gained from the debriefing can be used to develop further interdisciplinary team-training curriculum. Ultimately, simulation-based training can provide interdisciplinary teams an opportunity to work and learn together, a mechanism to promote and foster an environment of trust and collaboration.

Despite the high interest in using simulation to improve teamwork, few health care studies exist demonstrating that enhanced teamwork through simulation improves quality of care and patient outcomes. Neonatal simulation is still in its infancy; more research is needed to establish its effect and outcome in the real neonatal setting. Simulated environments, however, seem to be an effective training tool to enhance both individual and team performance in caring for the smallest and sickest of patients in a real-life setting, the NICU.

### *Scenarios*

Many patient simulators come with predefined scenarios for use in specialty areas such as the NICU. These case scenarios serve as the foundation for learning and are based on objectives for individual learners. Individualized scenarios can be developed to incorporate models for communication within interdisciplinary teams and between providers and parents. Knowing how to disclose errors and how to support families is a learned skill. Simulation-based training, along with well-designed patient scenarios, provide individuals and teams the opportunity to learn in a safe environment the skills needed to provide sensitive and compassionate care and communication to all families. Instructing care providers on how to communicate effectively and how to approach families sensitively can be incorporated successfully into well-designed simulation-based training programs for error and end-of-life disclosure.[73,74]

## INTERDISCIPLINARY TEAMS IN THE NEONATAL ICU

Multiple interdisciplinary teams exist in today's NICU (**Box 3**), and interactions among team members occur numerous times within a day. Teamwork, communication, and collaboration can be enhanced through the principles of CRM using simulation-based training and debriefing. Efficient and effective teams require leadership figures who model nonhierarchical communication, teamwork, and practice to optimize interactions among all team members, including nurses, physicians, families, pharmacists, therapists, social workers, chaplains, dieticians, and support staff. Nursing and physician leaders can support interdisciplinary teams by promoting a collaborative, respectful, nonhierarchical, and zero-tolerant culture.

**Box 3**
**Examples of interdisciplinary teams in the neonatal ICU**

Patient/family care team

Joint practice committee

Research committee

Evidence-based practice committee

Nutrition committee

Developmental care committee

Neonatal resuscitation committee

Quality improvement team

Bereavement/palliative care team

Patient safety team

Product/equipment evaluation

Education committee

The use of simulation and debriefing gives team members opportunities to be together and form relationships as they develop the cognitive, technical, and behavioral skills needed to function effectively. As team members from all disciplines spend time together and learn together, respect and trust for one another's judgment and expertise can develop. Respect and trust can influence how team members interact with one another and provide an environment in which every voice is heard and respected, regardless of whether everyone is in agreement. Senior nursing and physician leaders can work jointly to train and mentor junior staff, not only in the technical and cognitive skills of their job but also in behavioral skills by demonstrating how to approach and support families as a team when disclosing errors and communicating sensitive information. Outcome measures are needed to evaluate the effectiveness of simulation-based training and interdisciplinary teamwork and its impact on improved patient outcomes. Because teams make fewer mistakes than individuals,[57] team training and effective interdisciplinary teamwork in the NICU should be a priority in promoting patient safety.

## REFERENCES


1. Committee on Quality of Health Care in America. In: Kohn LT, Corrigan JM, Donaldson MS, editors. To err is human: building a safer health system. Washington (DC): National Academy Press; 2000.
2. Aspden P, the Committee on Institute of Medicine (U.S.). Patient safety: achieving a new standard for care. New York: National Academies P; 2004.
3. Agency for Healthcare Research and Quality. PSNet Patient Safety Network. Patient safety. Available at: http://psnet.ahrq.gov/glossary.aspx#p. Accessed September 15, 2008.
4. McClellan MB, McGinnis JM, Nabel EG, et al. Evidence-based medicine and the changing nature nature of health care. Washington, DC: National Academies Press; 2007.
5. Joseph A. The role of the physical environment in promoting health, safety, and effectiveness in the healthcare workplace. Research reports & papers. The Center for Health Design; Nov 2006. Available at: http://www.healthdesign.org/research/reports/workplace.php. Accessed September 15, 2008.
6. Hughes RG, editor. Patient safety and quality: an evidence-based handbook for nurses. vol. 1–3. Rockville (MD): Agency for Healthcare Research and Quality; 2008.
7. Luria JW, Muething SE, Schoettker PJ, et al. Reliability science and patient safety. Pediatr Clin North Am 2006;53(6):1121–33.
8. Mitchell PH. Defining patient safety and quality care. In: Hughes RG, editor. Patient safety and quality: an evidence-based handbook for nurses. vol. 1. Rockville (MD): Agency for Healthcare Research and Quality; 2008. p. 1–5.
9. Joint Commission. Behaviors that undermine a culture of safety. Sentinel event alert. 9 July 2008:40. Available at: http://www.jointcommission.org/sentinelevents/sentineleventalert/sea_40.htm. Accessed September 15, 2008.
10. Institute for Safe Medication Practices. Results from ISMP survey on workplace intimidation. ISMP. 2004. Available at: https://www.ismp.org/survey/surveyresults/survey0311.asp. Accessed September 15, 2008.
11. American Association of Critical-Care Nurses. American Association of Critical-Care Nurses standards for establishing and sustaining healthy work environments: a journey to excellence. Aliso Viejo (CA): American Associaton of Critical-Care Nurses; 2005.

12. American Nurses Association. Code of ethics for nurses with interpretive statements. Washington (DC): Author; 2001.
13. Page A, Board On Institute of Medicine (U.S.). Keeping patients safe: transforming the work environment of nurses. New York: National Academies P; 2003.
14. Committee on the Quality of Health Care in America. Crossing the quality chasm: a new health system for the 21st century. New York: National Academies P; 2001.
15. Greiner AC, Knebel E, editors. Health professions education: a bridge to quality. New York: National Academies Press; 2003.
16. Leape LL, Berwick DM. Five years after To Err is Human: what have we learned? JAMA 2005;293(19):2384–90.
17. Katzenbach JR, Smith DK. The wisdom of teams: creating the high-performance organization. Boston: McKinsey & Co; 1993.
18. Beaubien JM, Baker DP. The use of simulation for training teamwork skills in health care: how low can you go? Qual Saf Health Care 2004;13(Suppl 1):i51–6.
19. Jansen L. Collaborative and interdisciplinary health care teams: ready or not? J Prof Nurs 2008;24(4):218–27.
20. O'Daniel M, Rosenstein AH. Professional communication and team collaboration. In: Hughes RG, editor. Patient safety and quality: an evidence-based handbook for nurses. vol. 1. Rockville (MD): Agency for Healthcare Research and Quality; 2008. p. 271–84.
21. Roberts V, Perryman MM. Creating a culture for health care quality and safety. Health Care Manag (Fredrick) 2007;26(2):155–8.
22. Rushton CH. Respect in critical care: a foundational ethical principle. AACN Adv Crit Care 2007;18(2):149–56.
23. Weiss SJ, Davis HP. Validity and reliability of the Collaborative Practice Scales. Nurse Res 1985;34(5):299–305.
24. Henneman EA, Lee JL, Cohen JI. Collaboration: a concept analysis. J Adv Nurs 1995;21(1):103–9.
25. Silen-Lipponen M, Turrnen H, Tossavainen K. Collaboration in the operating room: the nurse's perspective. J Nurs Adm 2002;32(1):16–9.
26. Flin RG, Fletcher P, McGeorge, et al. Anaesthetists' attitudes to teamwork and safety. Anaesthesia 2005;58(3):233–42.
27. Azoulay E, Chevret S, Leleu G, et al. Half the families of intensive care unit patients experience inadequate communication with physicians. Crit Care Med 2000;28(8):3044–9.
28. SUPPORT Principal Investigators. A controlled trial to improve care for seriously ill hospitalized patients. The study to understand prognoses and preferences for outcomes and risks of treatments (SUPPORT). JAMA 1995;274(2):1591–8.
29. Institute for Family-Centered Care (FCC). Advancing the practice of patient-and family-centered care: how to get started. Bethesda (MD): Institute for Family-Centered Care; 2008.
30. American Academy of Pediatrics and the Committee on Hospital Care. Family-centered care and the pediatrician's role: policy statement. Washington (DC): American Academy of Pediatrics; 2003. reaffirmed 2007.
31. Joint Commission on Accreditation of Healthcare Organizations. The Joint Commission guide to improving staff communication. Oakbrook Terrace (IL): Joint Commission Resources; 2005.
32. Fein SP, Hilborne LH, Spiritus EM, et al. The many faces of error disclosure: a common set of elements and a definition. J Gen Intern Med 2007;22(6):755–61.
33. Mazor KM, Simon SR, Yood RA, et al. Health plan members' views about disclosure of medical errors. Ann Intern Med 2004;140(6):409–18.

34. Gallagher TH, Waterman AD, Ebers AG, et al. Patients' and physicians' attitudes regarding the disclosure of medical errors. JAMA 2003;289(8):1001–7.
35. Witman AB, Park DM, Hardin SB. How do patients want physicians to handle mistakes? A survey of internal medicine patients in an academic setting. Arch Intern Med 1996;156:2565–9.
36. Hobgood C, Peck CR, Gilbert B, et al. Medical errors—what and when: what do patients want to know? Acad Emerg Med 2002;9:1156–61.
37. Hobgood D, Tamayo-Sarver JH, Elms A, et al. Parental preferences for error disclosure, reporting, and legal action after medical error in the care of their children. Pediatrics 2005;116:1276–86.
38. Massachusetts Coalition for the Prevention of Medical Error. When things go wrong: responding to adverse events. Burlington (MA): Massachusetts Coalition for the Prevention of Medical Error; 2006.
39. Gallagher TH, Garbutt JM, Waterman AD, et al. Choosing your words carefully: how physicians would disclose harmful medical errors to patients. Arch Intern Med 2006;166(15):1585–93.
40. Leape LL. Full disclosure and apology—an idea whose time has come. Physician Exec 2006;32(2):16–8.
41. Sutcliffe K, Lewton E, Rosenthal M. Communication failures: an insidious contributor to medical mishaps. Acad Med 2004;79(2):186–94.
42. Rosenstein A. Nurse–physician relationships: impact on nurse satisfaction and retention. Am J Nurs 2002;102(6):26–34.
43. Rosenstein A, O'Daniel M. Disruptive behavior and clinical outcomes: perceptions of nurses and physicians. Am J Nurs 2005;105(1):54–64.
44. Helmreich RL. On error management: lessons from aviation. BMJ 2000;320(7237):781–5.
45. Sexton JB, Thomas EJ, Helmreich RL. Error, stress, and teamwork in medicine and aviation: cross sectional surveys. BMJ 2000;320(7237):745–9.
46. Salas E, Wilson KA, Murphy CD, et al. What crew resource management training will not do for patient safety: unless .... J Patient Saf 2007;3(2):62–4.
47. Hunt EA, Shilkofski NA, Stavroudis TA, et al. Simulation: translation to improved team performance. Anesthesiol Clin 2007;25(2):301–19.
48. McConaughey E. Crew resource management in healthcare: the evolution of teamwork training and MedTeams. J Perinat Neonatal Nurs 2008;22(2):96–104.
49. Thomas EJ, Taggart B, Crandell S, et al. Teaching teamwork during the Neonatal Resuscitation Program: a randomized trial. J Perinatol 2007;27(7):409–14.
50. Thomas EJ, Sexton JB, Lasky RE, et al. Teamwork and quality during neonatal care in the delivery room. J Perinatol 2006;26(3):163–9.
51. Halamek LP, Kaegi DM, Gaba DM, et al. Time for a new paradigm in pediatric medical education: teaching neonatal resuscitation in a simulated delivery room environment. Pediatrics 2000;106(4):e45. Available at: http://pediatrics.aappublications.org/cgi/content/full/106/4/e45. Accessed September 15, 2008.
52. Morey JC, Simon R, Jay GD, et al. Error reduction and performance improvement in the emergency department through formal teamwork training: evaluation results of the MedTeams project. Health Serv Res 2002;37(6):1553–81.
53. Eppich WJ, Brannen M, Hunt EA. Team training: implications for emergency and critical care pediatrics. Curr Opin Pediatr 2008;20(3):255–60.
54. France DJ, Leming-Lee S, Jackson T, et al. An observational analysis of surgical team compliance with perioperative safety practices after crew resource management training. Am J Surg 2008;195(4):546–53.

55. Makary MA, Sexton JB, Freischlag JA, et al. Operating room teamwork among physicians and nurses: teamwork in the eye of the beholder. J Am Coll Surg 2006;202(5):746–52.
56. Carthey J, de Leval MR, Wright DJ, et al. Behavioural markers of surgical excellence. Saf Sci 2003;41:409–25.
57. Baker DP, Gustafson S, Beaubien J, et al. Medical teamwork and patient safety: the evidence-based relation. Rockville (MD): Agency for Healthcare Research and Quality; April 2005. Available at: http://www.ahrq.gov/qual/medteam/. Accessed September 18, 2008.
58. Salas E, Wilson KA, Burke CS, et al. Does crew resource management training work? An update, an extension and some critical needs. Hum Factors 2006; 48(2):392–412.
59. Leonard MS, Graham S, Bonacum D. The human factor: the critical importance of effective teamwork and communication in providing safety care. Qual Saf Health Care 2004;13(Suppl 1):85–90.
60. Frissen MA, White SV, Byers JF. Handoffs: implications for nurses. In: Hughes RG, editor. Patient safety and quality: an evidence-based handbook for nurses. vol. 1. Rockville (MD): Agency for Healthcare Research and Quality; 2008. p. 285–332.
61. Joint Commission. 2008 National patient safety goals critical access hospital program. Jan 2008. Available at: http://www.jointcommission.org/patientsafety/nationalpatientsafetygoals/08_cah_npsgs.htm. Accessed September 15, 2008
62. Haig KM, Sutton S, Whittington J. SBAR: a shared mental model for improving communication between clinicians. Jt Comm J Qual Patient Saf 2006;32(3): 167–75.
63. Yaeger KA, Arafeh JM. Making the move from traditional neonatal education to simulation-based training. J Perinat Neonatal Nurs 2008;22(2):154–8.
64. Gaba DM. What does simulation add to teamwork training? Perspectives on safety. Available at: http://www.webmm.ahrq.gov/perspective.aspx?perspectiveid=20&%20searchstr=gaba+dm. Accessed on Sept 15, 2008.
65. Miller KK, Riley W, Davis S, et al. In situ-simulation: a method of experiential learning to promote safety and team behavior. J Perinat Neonatal Nurs 2008; 22(2):105–13.
66. Durham CF, Alden KR. Enhancing patient safety in nursing education through patient simulation. In: Hughes RG, editor. Patient safety and quality: an evidence-based handbook for nurses. vol. 1. Rockville (MD): Agency for Healthcare Research and Quality; 2008. p. 221–60.
67. Musson DM, Helmreich RL. Team training and resource management in health care: current issues and future directions. Harvard Health Policy Review 2004; 5:25–35.
68. The Accreditation Council for Graduate Medical Education. (ACGME). Simulation rehearsal. ACGME Bulletin Dec 2005. Available at: http://www.acgme.org/acwebsite/bulletin/bulletin12_05.pdf. Accessed September 24, 2008.
69. Halamek LP. The simulated delivery-room environment as the future modality for acquiring and maintaining skills in fetal and neonatal resuscitation. Semin Fetal Neonatal Med 2008;13(6):448–53.
70. Center for Advanced Pediatric & Perinatal Education (CAPE). CAPE videos—programs in action. Available at: http://www.cape.lpch.org/about/video/index.html. Accessed September 15, 2008.
71. Murphy AM, Halamek LP. Simulation-based training in neonatal resuscitation. NeoReviews 2005;6(11):489–92.

72. Hamman WR. The complexity of team training: what we have learned form aviation and its applications to medicine. Qual Saf Health Care 2004;13(Supp 1):72–9.
73. Wayman KI, Yaeger KA, Sharek PJ, et al. JHQ 198 simulation-based medical error disclosure training for pediatric healthcare professionals. July-Aug. 2007. Available at: http://www.nahq.org/journal/ce/article.html?article_id=283. Accessed September 15, 2008.
74. Mosher PJ, Murphy AA, Anderson JM, et al. Death, dying and delivering bad news: simulation-based training improves the skills and confidence of medical students. Presented at Pediatric Academic Societies/Society for Pediatric Research Annual Meeting. San Francisco, CA; May 1–4, 2004.
75. Joint Commission. Sentinel event glossary of terms. Available at: http://www.jointcommission.org/SentinelEvents/se_glossary.htm. Accessed September 15, 2008.
76. Patterson ES, Roth EM, Woods DD, et al. Handoff strategies in settings with high consequences for failure: lessons for health care operations. Int J Qual Health Care 2004;16(2):125–32.

# Nutritional Support of Very Low Birth Weight Newborns

Georgia Ditzenberger, NNP-BC, PhD[a,b]

**KEYWORDS**

- VLBW infant, newborn • Premature newborn
- Postnatal growth restriction

Nutritional support to promote optimal postnatal growth for very low birth weight (VLBW) newborns less than 1500 g at birth during the initial prolonged hospitalization is a significant issue. During the past 4 decades, improvements in such areas as thermoregulation, ventilatory support, and fluid and electrolyte management have made it possible for more VLBW newborns survive to discharge from neonatal intensive care units (NICUs). VLBW newborns spend 2 to 3 months in the NICU, maturing to 35 to 42 weeks of postmenstrual age (PMA) in preparation for discharge. The National Institute of Child Health and Human Development Neonatal Network reported that although intrauterine growth restriction was present in 22% of VLBW newborns at birth, 91% of newborns demonstrated postnatal growth restriction by 36 weeks of PMA.[1] Growth restriction, intrauterine and postnatal, is defined as body weight less than the 10th percentile on reference growth curves.

Conditions with potential confounding effects on postnatal growth include genetic conditions inhibiting growth; bronchopulmonary dysplasia* (BPD; oxygen requirement after 36 weeks of gestation); small for gestational age (SGA) status at birth; late-onset sepsis; neurologic conditions, including intraventricular hemorrhage (IVH), hydrocephaly, microcephaly, and periventricular leukomalacia (PVL); patent ductus arteriosus (PDA) requiring intervention; and gastrointestinal conditions, such as feeding intolerance, necrotizing enterocolitis (NEC), or short gut syndrome.[1,2]

The persistent growth deficit in VLBW newborns is associated with the inadequacy of protein and energy intake during the initial hospitalization when controlling for potential confounding effects.[1,3–9] Inadequate protein and energy intake may account for 45% to 50% of the postnatal growth restriction seen by the end of the initial

* Bronchopulmonary dysplasia is often used interchangeably with chronic lung disease. Current literature is favoring a return to the term *bronchopulmonary dysplasia* over *chronic lung disease* because of the confusion with chronic lung diseases of older adults not related to premature birth.

[a] Division of Neonatology, Department of Pediatrics, University of Wisconsin School of Medicine and Public Health, Madison, WI, USA
[b] Neonatal Advanced Practice Nursing and Research, Meriter Hospital, Inc., 202 S. Park Street, Madison, WI 53515-1596, USA
*E-mail address:* ditzeg@pediatrics.wisc.edu

Crit Care Nurs Clin N Am 21 (2009) 181–194
doi:10.1016/j.ccell.2009.01.005 ccnursing.theclinics.com
0899-5885/09/$ – see front matter 

hospitalization, with the remainder attributable to effects from underlying conditions.[8,10] Recent changes in commercially prepared formulas and human milk fortifiers are associated with a reduction in postnatal growth restriction from 97% in 2001 to 91% in 2007.[1,11] Although this reduction in postnatal growth restriction in the past decade is significant, the problem clearly persists.

This article reviews the concepts involved in the nutritional support of VLBW newborns, including definitions and discussions of growth, optimal postnatal growth, body composition, initial weight loss of VLBW newborns, growth expectations, growth assessment tools used during the postnatal period, the relation between inadequate nutrition and neurodevelopment, the relation between protein intake and cognitive outcome, postnatal nutrition balance, the potential for programming of future adult-onset chronic conditions, a review of fetal nutritional intake, and current recommendations for nutritional support of VLBW newborns.

## GROWTH

Growth is "the progressive development of a living thing, especially the process by which the body reaches its point of complete physical development...from infancy to maturity involves great changes in body size and appearance...not a steady [process]; at some times growth occurs rapidly, at others slowly. Individual patterns of growth vary widely because of differences in heredity and environment."[12] Fetal, neonatal, and infant periods of the human life cycle are such times of rapid growth. Heredity plays an important part in determining the potential for growth (eg, genetic potential), but environment, which supports access to adequate nutrients for growth, also is important to sustain growth to genetic potential.

## OPTIMAL POSTNATAL GROWTH

Optimal growth for VLBW newborns during the postnatal period to 40 weeks of PMA is currently defined by the American Academy of Pediatrics as approximating "the rate of growth and composition of weight gain for a normal fetus of the same postmenstrual age."[13] Therefore, assessing VLBW newborn growth seems to be straightforward (ignoring, for the moment, the composition of weight gain); if one has access to a fetal growth chart, one can compare VLBW newborn measurements to determine the attainment of optimal growth.

Gestational age is determined by the "best obstetric estimate," a combination of the first day of the last menstrual period; physical examination of the mother; prenatal ultrasonography; and history, if any, of assisted reproduction.[14] Newborns are typically measured soon after birth and determined to be appropriate for gestational age (AGA) if measurements of head circumference, length, and weight are within the 10th and 90th percentile curves for fetal growth, SGA if at or below the 10th percentile curve, or large for gestational age if at or above the 90th percentile curve.[15] Symmetric growth is determined when all measurements are within the same percentile curves; for example, symmetric SGA is when measurements for head circumference, length, and weight are of the 10th percentile curve or less. Asymmetric growth is defined when one or more measurements are in differing percentile curves.[16]

## BODY COMPOSITION

The clinical assessment of the distribution of weight in fat mass and lean muscle mass, or body composition, may be a cursory visual assessment and not an accurate or objective summation of body composition. Adequate growth to genetic potential implies lean mass accumulation and brain volume development in addition to generalized somatic growth and fat deposition to maintain body composition comparable to that of a fetus of similar gestation.[13] Weight-for-length is helpful for assessment of growth symmetry in body composition for stable older VLBW newborns. Ponderal indices have been used to determine fetal and neonatal body composition to assess for growth restriction and may be of use for body composition assessment during the postnatal period of VLBW newborns.[17–19]

VLBW newborns may need greater weight gains than the estimated fetal weight accretion rate of 14.4 to 16.1 g/kg/d to overcome the effect of initial weight loss and the prolonged period before regaining birth weight. Initial weight loss is expected for all newborns regardless of gestational age and, until the past decade, had been thought to be primarily attributable to extracellular fluid loss. Up to 50% of the initial weight loss for VLBW newborns may be attributable to the loss of endogenous glycogen and lipid stores and lean tissue mass that have been used to meet metabolic energy demands in the absence of adequate nutrition, however.[20]

## WEIGHT LOSS IN FIRST DAYS OF LIFE

Typically, healthy term newborns lose up to 5% to 7% of body weight in the first days of life, regain to birth weight by 7 days of life, and then begin expected weight gains of 30 g/d during the initial infant growing phase to 3 months of age.[21,22] VLBW newborns lose a greater percentage of birth weight, up to 15%, with decreasing gestational age at birth and may take an average of 2.5 weeks to regain birth weight. Extremely low birth weight newborns weighing less than 1000 g at birth could potentially manifest up to 20% weight loss and may take up to 3 to 4 weeks to regain birth weight.[8,23,24] The prolonged period under birth weight during the postnatal stage of VLBW newborns increases the gap between expected growth on the standard growth curves to the point where, by 32 weeks of PMA, VLBW newborns can weigh 35% to 41% less than newborns who are 32 weeks' gestation at birth.[23] Achieving genetic growth potential, growth based on heredity, is thwarted by the lack of environmental support, which, in this case, is nutritional support in the NICU. The longer it takes to regain birth weight, the more difficult it is to regain an optimal growth pattern based on genetic growth potential, including increases in length and head circumference measurements, resulting in postnatal growth restriction.

## GROWTH EXPECTATIONS

Growth expectations for VLBW newborns are the optimal gains in growth measurements that meet the "normal" incremental increases depicted on growth curves in addition to any catch-up increases required to regain an optimal growth pattern. Although it is common to discuss growth expectations of VLBW newborns in terms of weight gains, gains in head circumference and lengths are just as necessary to determine optimal growth. Head circumference has a close relation to the growth of brain volume.[20,25,26] Heird[27] reported that the "critical" period for brain growth spans at least the first 18 months of life for VLBW newborns and that correction of early nutritional shortfalls during this time may avoid neurodevelopmental outcome deficits associated with VLBW newborns. Length in comparison to weight gives a good indication of body composition, if accurately measured.[28]

To date, recommendations for expected weight gains to achieve optimal growth for VLBW newborns are not defined beyond attempting to regain the growth percentile curve at which the newborn started. The best estimate of optimal daily weight gains to achieve this goal is currently recommended to begin with 15 to 20 g/kg/d and adjust caloric intake in response to the newborn's daily weight gains averaged over 3 to 5 days.[29] The expected gain in head circumference for 24 to 40 weeks is 0.1 to 0.6 cm/wk; for length, it is 0.69 to 0.75 cm/wk.[20]

## GROWTH ASSESSMENT TOOLS

Anthropometric measurements are the most direct tools used to determine patterns in growth. The most commonly used anthropometric measurements are weight, length, and head circumference. Growth velocities are the incremental changes of these three measurements either daily, as in the case of weight, or weekly, as for length and head circumference. Weight gains, weight gain velocity, and head circumferences are primary end points of research of postnatal growth of VLBW newborns.[2–5,7,25,30–33]

Body weight is the most commonly performed measurement and the most readily accepted as an accurate determinant of growth in all pediatric populations.[34,35] Weight fluctuations are predominant, with hydration status changes, particularly in the first 1 to 2 weeks of life. After the first 1 to 2 weeks of life, weight changes are accepted to be the reflection of nutritional support when interpreted together with other anthropometric parameters, such as length and head circumference.[2,3,7,9,29,32,36–39] Errors in weight accuracy can occur with failure to zero the scale, not allowing the scale to stabilize, not removing clothing or diapers, difficulty in preventing attached lines and leads from touching the scale bed, and failure to compare the weight with previously recorded weights.[40]

Length measurement is most typically the crown-to-heel (crown-heel) measurement. At best, length is measured weekly by experienced personnel with a length board specific for premature infants, such as the O'Leary Premie Length Board (Ellard Instrumentation LTD, Seattle, Washington). Accuracy in length measurement is confounded by physical characteristics, such as temporary head molding caused by delivery or positioning, or lower extremity contractions. Clothing, especially diapers, hampers the ability to obtain full body length.

Head circumference, also known as occipital-frontal circumference, is determined by applying paper or plasticized paper measurement tape firmly around the head above the supraorbital ridges, over the most prominent part of the frontal bulge interiorly, and over the part of the occiput giving the maximum circumference.[32] Head circumference measurements are used serially to track increasing hydrocephalus or worsening microcephaly and for growth response. Care must be taken in interpretation of changes, however, because the measurements also reflect generalized scalp edema, molding from delivery or positioning, or other aspects of clinical condition.

## GROWTH CURVE CHARTS

Typical growth curve charts with weight, length, and head circumference, which are used in the NICU to establish growth patterns and in current research, are generally those based on fetal growth and, less frequently, on the growth of former VLBW newborns. Controversy prevails over the assessment of optimal growth for VLBW newborns during the postnatal period, particularly whether the growth of VLBW newborns should be assessed using fetal growth curves based on birth measurements or on the postnatal growth of data collected from actual VLBW newborns.[5,41]

Fetal growth curves are the "gold standard" for VLBW newborn growth because the curves reflect the growth that VLBW newborns might have experienced in utero at similar gestations.[9,13,29,32,41] Reference charts based on VLBW newborns' growth parameters reflect slower growth patterns and much lower average measurements of weight, length, and head circumference than the gold standard of fetal growth.[9,13,29,32,39,42]

Arguments for the use of charts based on former VLBW newborns' growth patterns center on the question of whether growth of VLBW newborns should be a reflection of fetal growth or if another growth pattern is more appropriate for postnatal growth assessment.[8,32,41,43] Recent studies of newborns with postnatal growth similar to growth curves based on VLBW newborns, such as the chart by Ehrenkranz and colleagues,[24] and followed through to school age reported neurologic and physical deficits consistent with earlier findings.[11,44–47] Because postnatal growth restriction is associated with poorer outcomes, it does not seem appropriate to use growth curves based on the actual postnatal growth of VLBW newborns as references for the assessment of current VLBW newborns.

Babson and Benda[48] developed the first growth chart incorporating fetal and newborn birth data through 1 year of age for weight, head circumference, and length measurements into one growth curve chart. Called the "Fetal-Infant Growth Graph," these growth curves have been commonly used.[33] The graph's strengths included the combined fetal and newborn data, which extended its usefulness, and the fact that it was accessible during the postnatal period to assess premature newborn growth. Limitations include an exclusively white newborn sample with small subsets for each gestational age derived from data that were 15 years old at the time of development.[48] Still, it was a landmark work, which provided many NICU practitioners with a practical tool for assessing premature newborn growth during the postnatal period.

The updated Fetal-Infant Growth Graph includes meta-analysis results of data from published studies performed in Canada, Sweden, New South Wales, the United States (including studies by the United States Centers for Disease Control and Prevention), Norway, and the United Kingdom. The data, from studies done from 1982 to 2002, include a combined ethnically diverse sample of fetuses and newborns from 22 to 40 weeks of gestation and term newborns to 50 weeks of PMA, with weekly increments for weight, head circumference, and length. The graph reflects a third-trimester fetal weight accretion rate of 14.4 to 16.1 g/kg/d from 26 to 40 weeks.[33]

## RELATION BETWEEN INADEQUATE NUTRITION AND NEURODEVELOPMENT

Multiple studies have examined the effects of early malnutrition on central nervous system (CNS) development in experimental animal models and after periods of starvation or low intakes of energy or essential nutrient requirements in human infants and children. Reduction of nutrition support during fetal and neonatal life and during infancy can cause profound effects on the somatic growth and development of organ structure or function, especially of the brain and CNS, causing decreased body and brain growth.[49] Adequate nutrition plays a prominent role in supporting growth to genetic potential during such times of rapid growth and development.

Inadequate nutrition as a cause of postnatal growth restriction is of great concern because of the growing body of evidence supporting that undernutrition during critical periods of brain growth results in irreversible lifelong neurodevelopmental deficits.[7,50–53] Recent results from follow-up studies indicate that if improved head circumference measurements, reflecting brain growth in the absence of CNS abnormalities, do not occur within the first 3 to 8 months of postnatal life, there is not likely to be further "catch-up" head circumference growth.[42,45,46,54,55]

There may be a sensitive period for head circumference growth and inferred increasing brain volume between 30 weeks of PMA and 6 months of corrected age.[46] Limperopoulos and colleagues[56] demonstrated a period of rapid cerebellar growth between 28 weeks of PMA and term with serial MRI brain scans of 129 VLBW newborns during initial hospitalization. The cerebellar volume of the VLBW newborns at term PMA was significantly smaller than that of healthy term newborn equivalents. Multiple factors were associated with decreased cerebellar development and the resultant decreased brain volume, particularly lower gestational age at birth, severity of condition, and slower changes in postnatal growth parameters of head circumference and weight.[56]

## RELATION BETWEEN PROTEIN INTAKE AND COGNITIVE OUTCOME

Cautious nutritional support given to VLBW newborns during the first days to weeks of life results in severe deficits in all nutritional components, particularly protein.[7,29,57] Deficits in protein may reach up to 30 g/kg over the course of the initial hospital stay for VLBW newborns.[8] Protein accretion is at its greatest between 22 and 32 weeks of fetal age, indicating a heightened fetal need for protein during peak cerebellar development.[29,50,51,58] This dichotomy between fetal protein accretion rates and postnatal protein intakes for VLBW newborns may be a key factor in the decreased brain growth of VLBW newborns manifesting postnatal growth restriction. Protein intakes close to the fetal accretion rate may still need to be the goal of postnatal nutrition to meet the increased requirement of VLBW newborn for protein synthesis, growth, and neuronal development.

Protein and energy intake deficiencies lead to decreased cell division and myelination in the developing brain, resulting in lower brain volume and minimal head circumference growth, with a strong association with poor cognitive, motor, and behavioral outcomes.[26,45,46,55,56,59] Arslanoglu and colleagues[2] reported a significant correlation between improved head circumference growth, inferring greater brain volume, and enteral protein intake between 3.6 and 4.0 g/kg/d.

Motor, cognitive, and behavioral consequences of postnatal undernutrition are difficult to differentiate from other factors that also may contribute to altered neurodevelopment, such as genetics, IVH, PVL, and BPD. Several longitudinal studies of VLBW newborns have demonstrated neurodevelopmental sequelae not totally accounted for by factors other than postnatal undernutrition.[8,32,44,53,60,61]

A growing body of evidence supports the predictor value of early postnatal growth for VLBW newborns during initial postnatal hospitalization and long-term neurodevelopmental outcome when other factors are taken into consideration.[53,55] AGA VLBW newborns who remain on the same growth curve through to discharge have better neurodevelopmental outcome at 24 months of age than do VLBW newborns who are of AGA at birth but drop to lower than the 10th percentile growth curve (SGA) at discharge.[32,44,52,53,56,60,62,63]

## POTENTIAL PROGRAMMING FOR FUTURE ADULT ONSET OF CHRONIC DISEASE

Growing evidence suggests that rapid growth during the postnatal period of VLBW newborns, often called "catch-up growth," may stimulate alterations in metabolism, hormonal output, and distribution of cardiac output, resulting in "programming" for development of central obesity, diabetes, and cardiovascular disease in later adulthood.[42,53] This type of programming may also occur because of changes in metabolism that result from alterations made during periods of undernutrition during the fetal period or early infancy.[42] VLBW newborns typically experience undernutrition during the first days to weeks of life, followed by catch-up growth that extends beyond discharge into the first year of life.[42,43,53,64–66]

On first consideration, there seems to be a dilemma between the need to prevent postnatal growth restriction associated with poor neurodevelopmental outcome by increased postnatal growth, or catch-up growth, and the need to prevent programming for later adult-onset health diseases by preventing rapid postnatal growth. It may be that early nutritional support with aggressive administration of nutrients in appropriate amounts for postnatal growth may reduce postnatal growth restriction and diminish the necessity for later increased nutrient supplementation to provide for rapid catch-up of growth.[54]

## POSTNATAL NUTRITION BALANCE

Aggressive postnatal nutrition must not just focus on increased protein intake. Adequate protein metabolism and synthesis require appropriate protein energy balance. Neuronal development also requires sufficient fatty acid accretion for neuronal myelination and energy needs. Thus, nutritional support to minimize postnatal growth restriction and maximize optimal neurodevelopmental outcome must take into consideration the amount of each nutrient, with less emphasis on glucose and fat and increased protein amounts that approximate fetal intakes and yield appropriate lean-to-fat body mass accretion from birth to discharge of initial hospitalization.[29,53,57,67]

VLBW newborns seem to tolerate higher protein intakes, with limited evidence for minimal metabolic adverse sequelae. More research is needed to determine the amount and duration of higher protein intakes and if providing differing amounts of protein based on body weight is beneficial in support of growth with body composition distributions closer to those of fetal and healthy term newborn growth patterns.

Improved nutrition support for ongoing growth from birth throughout hospitalization, with initiation of intravenous nutrition containing "appropriate" nutrient components immediately after birth, followed by complete enteral nutrition, may decrease the later catch-up growth period and reduce programming effects for later adult-onset health diseases.[68,69] In this respect, postnatal growth differs from catch-up growth in that the increases in growth are supported throughout the initial postnatal period rather than development of postnatal growth restriction followed by a period of rapid catch-up growth.

There is strong negative evidence associating decreased protein intake with poor neurodevelopmental outcome and minimal but growing positive evidence to support that increasing protein intake may improve neurodevelopmental outcome. There is encouraging but limited evidence of the short-term effect of protein intakes of 3.6 to 4.0 g/kg/d on head circumference and weight with improved neurodevelopmental outcome through 2 years, but these findings fall short of the long-term evidence needed to show continued positive neurologic outcome without other adverse sequelae.

## FETAL ENERGY, FAT, GLUCOSE, AND PROTEIN INTAKES

Estimates of third-trimester fetal energy requirements are 90 to 100 kcal/kg/d to support weight gains of 14.4 to 16.1 g/kg/d and are primarily met through metabolism of glucose, lactate, and amino acids.[21] The fetal fat accretion rate between 26 and 30 weeks of gestation is 1 to 1.8 g/kg/d; by 36 to 40 weeks of gestation, the rate is 1.6 to 3.4 g/kg/d.[70]

Glucose is the primary carbohydrate source used in fetal and premature infant nutrition. It is also the primary energy source for the brain and an important carbon source for synthesis of nonessential amino acids and fatty acids.[21,36,71,72] Glucose is delivered to the fetus by way of the placenta at a rate that matches fetal energy use rates of 4 to 6 mg/kg$^{-1}$/min$^{-1}$ and is the major source of energy intake, accounting for 80%; protein meets most of the remaining 20% fetal energy need.[21]

The fetal protein accretion rate depends directly on the rate of fetal somatic accruement and on organ and brain growth. The third trimester, beginning at approximately 26 weeks of gestation, is significant for rapid increases in somatic and brain growth and reflects increased fetal protein accretion and use. During this time, the fetal protein accretion rate is estimated to be 3.6 to 4.8 g/kg/d.[73]

## RECOMMENDATIONS FOR ENERGY, FAT, GLUCOSE, AND PROTEIN INTAKES FOR VERY LOW BIRTH WEIGHT NEWBORNS

Nutritional recommendations to support optimal growth are based on estimated fetal intakes and evidence from limited research.[71] Historically, research in the 1980s by neonatal pioneers, such as Kashyap, Heird, and others, established enteral energy intake recommendations for VLBW newborns at 110 to 135 kcal/kg/d to manifest weight gains averaging 15 to 20 g/kg/d.[21,72,74] The increase in postnatal energy requirement compared with fetal energy requirement is explained, in part, by the increased caloric expenditure for thermoregulation, digestion, cardiovascular maintenance, and other physiologic processes.[72,74,75] Parenteral energy intake is estimated to be 90 to 110 kcal/kg/d, slightly less than enteral energy intake because of the absence of caloric expenditure for digestion, absorption, and elimination.[21,76]

Energy intakes include the caloric contributions from fat, carbohydrate (glucose), and protein intakes unless specified otherwise.[72] Often, the terms *nonprotein energy intake* and *energy intake* are not specifically defined and are used interchangeably.[13,65,72,74] Fat yields approximately 9 kcal/g, glucose yields approximately 3.4 kcal/g, and protein yields approximately 4 kcal/g.[77,78] At the bedside, for example, parenteral nutrition for a 1000-g VLBW newborn at a rate of 150 mL/kg/d with 14% dextrose (73 kcal), protein at a rate of 3.5 g/kg/d (14 kcal), and fat at a rate of 3 g/kg/d (27 kcal) would be 114 kcal/kg/d with, or 100 kcal/kg/d without, the energy from protein added into the calculations. Given the relatively low contribution of protein intake (~12% in the example) to total energy intake and the fact that most protein intake is potentially used for lean muscle mass accumulation and brain growth rather than for energy, making the distinction between nonprotein energy intake and energy intake may not be important for daily discussions at the bedside. The distinction may make a difference in research accuracy and interpretation, however.

Current recommendations for VLBW newborn postnatal intake of fat is 1 to 3 g/kg/d at initiation, increasing to as high as 7.2 g/kg/d, for energy, neuronal myelination, and fat mass accretion.[13,70,71] Research is ongoing regarding whether the fat profile for parenteral and enteral nutrition should be closer to fetal sources or breast milk and if fat intake should exceed 3.5 g/kg/d, which is closer to the fetal accretion rate through the third trimester and, theoretically, supports appropriate development of body composition.[70,71]

Current recommendations for VLBW newborn postnatal intake of glucose intake match the fetal use rate soon after birth with 4 to 6 mg/kg$^{-1}$/min$^{-1}$ (7.5–8.4 g/kg/d) and increasing gradually to a maximum of 12 mg/kg$^{-1}$/min$^{-1}$ (17 g/kg/d). There is limited research to substantiate the current recommendations for carbohydrate, other than some evidence that carbohydrate is more effective than fat in promoting nitrogen retention in premature infants. There are concerns about long-term effects of early high-carbohydrate intakes, which support the restriction of glucose loads to 12 mg/kg$^{-1}$/min$^{-1}$ or less to reduce disproportionate body composition (ie, greater fat than lean body mass stores). As a result, recommendations for carbohydrate intakes for VLBW newborns are theoretic, balanced between the limited evidence of benefit and the potential long-term effects, until more research provides supportive evidence to determine appropriate values.[71]

Current protein intake recommendations for VLBW newborns vary from 2.25 to 3.6 g per 100 kcal (2.7–4.3 g/kg/d). This should be accompanied by concomitant nonprotein energy intakes of 90 to 100 kcal/kg/d if receiving parenteral nutrition or 110 to 130 kcal/kg/d if receiving enteral nutrition.[9,21,38,57,59,71,74,76,79] Parenteral protein intakes vary from 1 to 3.5 g per 100 kcal based on the current practices in individual NICUs. Commercial premature newborn formulas and human milk fortifiers delivered at a rate of 24 cal/oz deliver 2.8 to 3.2 g per 100 kcal (3.4 to 3.8 g/kg/d) when enteral caloric intake is 120 kcal/kg/d.

## PROTEIN-TO-ENERGY RATIO

Protein intake is discussed in terms of the protein-to-energy ratio (P:E) in grams per 100 kcal and in g/kg/d rather than g/d because of the dependency of weight distribution on the P:E of the nutrition provided to VLBW newborns. Although energy and protein intakes are considered independently in terms of g/kg/d, protein intakes should be determined based on the amount of concomitant energy intake, and vice versa, to provide adequate energy substrate for metabolic expenditure, maximize the rate of weight gain, and promote appropriate body composition. Nitrogen retention resulting in lean body mass increases with increasing protein intake; increasing energy intake also increases nitrogen retention with adequate protein intakes.[71,74,80–82] If energy intakes are increased without increasing protein intakes, however, increased storage of fat versus lean tissue occurs.[71,72,74] Conversely, if protein intakes exceed adequate concurrent energy intakes, the potential for adverse events, such as increased oxygen consumption and carbon dioxide release, or lactic acid buildup could occur.[78,83]

When discussing protein intakes without consideration of the P:E relation, the amount of protein, similar to glucose and fat intake, is presented in terms of g/kg/d rather than g/d. This custom is used to reduce confusion in using lengthy graphs depicting nutrient intake recommendations for each body weight and to provide a standard of comparison between protein, glucose, and fat intakes. For example, protein intake a rate of 3.5 g/kg/d for a 1500-g newborn is 5.3 g/d; for a 690-g newborn, it is 2.4 g/d. Both newborns are getting different total protein intake in g/d but receiving the same relative protein intake in g/kg/d.

It is difficult to achieve current recommendations for nutritional intake during the immediate postnatal period. Embleton and colleagues,[8] in a prospective observational study, compared desired dietary requirements with actual protein and energy intakes of 105 premature newborns with birth weights of 1750 g or less. The desired nutritional support established in the NICU was defined as energy intake at 120 kcal/kg/d and protein intake at 3 g/kg/d. Embleton and colleagues[8] calculated daily deficits in energy and protein by subtracting actual intake from calculated desired intake. The calculated deficits by 1 week of age for VLBW newborns 31 weeks or greater of gestation were a protein deficit of 12 $\pm$ 4 g and an energy deficit of 335 $\pm$ 86 kcal ($P<.001$). Newborns 30 weeks or less of gestation showed a protein deficit of 14 $\pm$ 4 g and an energy deficit of 405 $\pm$ 92 kcal ($P<.001$). By the end of 5 weeks, VLBW newborns 31 weeks or greater of gestation accrued a protein deficit of 13 $\pm$ 4 g and a nonprotein energy deficit of 382 $\pm$ 86 kcal ($P<.001$). At the end of 5 weeks VLBW newborns at 30 weeks or less of gestation showed a protein deficit of 23 $\pm$ 4 g and a nonprotein energy deficit of 813 $\pm$ 92 kcal (*P*<.001).

Deficits in protein and energy occurred in spite of the best intent of the NICU nutritional management team. The deficits in protein and energy intakes were most severe for infants at 30 weeks or less gestation. For all VLBW newborns, the deficits are difficult to surmount in the postnatal period of hospitalization, regardless of the severity of the cumulative deficit.

## SUMMARY

Postnatal growth restriction is associated with inadequate protein and energy intakes. Current recommendations for nutritional support of VLBW newborns rely on the estimates of fetal energy, fat, glucose, and protein intakes for the third trimester of pregnancy and on limited evidence from research. It is difficult to achieve the recommended amounts, particularly for protein, because of the physical limitations of VLBW newborns during the immediate postnatal period. The nutritional needs of VLBW newborns may differ from those of a fetus of similar gestational age, and protein requirements may be greater to account for consistent promotion of growth in the extrauterine environment. It is thus important to continue to seek the most appropriate nutritional support to promote optimal growth toward the genetic potential of VLBW newborns.

## REFERENCES

1. Fanaroff AA, Stoll BJ, Wright LL, et al. Trends in neonatal morbidity and mortality for very low birthweight infants. Am J Obstet Gynecol 2007;196(2):147, e141–8.
2. Arslanoglu S, Moro GE, Ziegler EE. Adjustable fortification of human milk fed to preterm infants: does it make a difference? J Perinatol 2006;26(10):614–21.
3. Bertino E, Coscia A, Mombro M, et al. Postnatal weight increase and growth velocity of very low birthweight infants. Arch Dis Child Fetal Neonatal Ed 2006; 91:349–56.
4. Clark RH, Thomas P, Peabody J. Extrauterine growth restriction remains a serious problem in prematurely born neonates. Pediatrics 2003;111(5):986–90.
5. Cooke R. Postnatal growth in preterm infants. In: Thureen PJ, Hay WW, editors. Neonatal nutrition and metabolism. 2nd edition. New York: Cambridge University Press; 2006.
6. de Boo HA, Harding JE. Protein metabolism in preterm infants with particular reference to intrauterine growth restriction. Arch Dis Child Fetal Neonatal Ed 2007;92(4):F315–9.
7. De Curtis M, Rigo J. Extrauterine growth restriction in very low birthweight infants. Acta Paediatr 2004;93:1563–8.
8. Embleton NE, Pang N, Cooke RJ. Postnatal malnutrition and growth retardation: an inevitable consequence of current recommendations in preterm infants? Pediatrics 2001;107(2):270–4.
9. Fenton T, Sauve RS. Higher versus lower protein intake in formula-fed low birth weight infants (review). Cochrane Database Syst Rev 2006;(4):1–33. CD003959.
10. Maggio L, Cota F, Lauriola V, et al. Effects of high versus standard early protein intake on growth of extremely low birth weight infants. J Pediatr Gastroenterol Nutr 2007;44:124–9.
11. Lemons JA, Bauer CR, Oh W, et al. Very low birth weight outcomes of the National Institute of Child Health and Human Development Neonatal Research Network, January 1995 through December 1996. Pediatrics 2001;107(1):e1–7.

12. Miller BF, Keane CB. Encyclopedia and dictionary of medicine and nursing. Philadelphia: W.B.Saunders Company; 1972.
13. Kleinman RE. Pediatric nutrition handbook. 5th edition. Elkhorn (IL): American Academy of Pediatrics; 2004.
14. Committee on Fetus and Newborn A. Age terminology during the perinatal period. Pediatrics 2004;114:1362–4.
15. Anderson DM. Nutritional implications of premature birth, birth weight, and gestational age classification. In: Groh-Wargo S, Thompson M, Cox JH, editors. Nutritional care for high-risk newborns. 3rd edition. Chicago: Precept Press, Inc.; 2000.
16. Zerzan J. Intrauterine growth retardation (IUGR) and small for gestational age (SGA): implications for growth, outcome, and nutrition management. Nutrition Focus 2004;19(4):1–8.
17. Burkhardt T, Schaffer L, Zimmermann R, et al. Newborn weight charts underestimate the incidence of low birthweight in preterm infants. Am J Obstet Gynecol 2008;199(2):139. e1–6.
18. Khoury MJ, Berg CJ, Calle EE. The ponderal index in term newborn siblings. Am J Epidemiol 1990;132(3):576–83.
19. Vintzileos AM, Lodeiro JG, Feinstein SJ, et al. Value of fetal ponderal index in predicting growth retardation. Obstet Gynecol 1986;67(4):584–8.
20. Katrine K. Anthropometric assessment. In: Groh-Wargo S, Thompson M, Cox JH, editors. Nutritional care for high-risk newborns. 3rd edition. Chicago: Precept Press, Inc.; 2000.
21. Blackburn ST. Maternal, fetal, and neonatal physiology: a clinical perspective. 3rd edition. Philadelphia: Elsevier/Saunders; 2007.
22. Dewey KG, Nommsen-Rivers LA, Heinig MJ, et al. Risk factors for suboptimal infant breastfeeding behavior, delayed onset of lactation, and excess neonatal weight loss. Pediatrics 2003;112(3):607–19.
23. Bhatia J. Post-discharge nutrition of preterm infants. J Perinatol 2005;25(Suppl 2): S15–6.
24. Ehrenkranz RA, Younes N, Lemons JA, et al. Longitudinal growth of hospitalized very low birth weight infants. Pediatrics 1999;104(2):280–97.
25. Brandt I, Sticker EJ, Lentze MJ. Catch-up growth of head circumference of very low birth weight, small for gestational age preterm infants and mental development to adulthood. J Pediatr 2003;142(5):463–70.
26. Poindexter BB, Langer JC, Dusick AM, et al. Early provision of parenteral amino acids in extremely low birth weight infants: relation to growth and neurodevelopmental outcome. J Pediatr 2006;148:300–5.
27. Heird WC. The importance of early nutritional management of low-birthweight infants. Pediatr Rev 1999;20(9):e43–4.
28. Wood NS, Costeloe K, Gibson AT, et al. The EPICure study: growth and associated problems in children born at 25 weeks of gestational age or less. Arch Dis Child Fetal Neonatal Ed 2003;88(6):F492–500.
29. Hay W. Nutritional requirements of the very preterm infant. Acta Paediatr 2005;94: 37–46.
30. Bhatia J, Rassin DK, Cerreto MC, et al. Effect of protein/energy ratio on growth and behavior of premature infants: preliminary findings. J Pediatr 1991;119: 103–10.
31. de Onis M, Garza C, Onyango AW, et al. Comparison of the WHO child growth standards and the CDC 2000 growth charts. J Nutr 2007;137(1):144–8.
32. Ehrenkranz RA, Dusick AM, Vohr B, et al. Network Research Network NICHD. Growth in the neonatal intensive care unit influences neurodevelopmental and

growth outcomes of extremely low birth weight infants. Pediatrics 2006;117: 1253–61.
33. Fenton T. A new growth chart for preterm babies: Babson and Benda's chart updated with recent data and a new format. BMC Pediatr 2003;3(1):13–22.
34. Feucht S. Assessment of growth, part 1: equipment, technique and growth charts. Nutrition Focus 2000;15(2):1–8.
35. Trahms C, Feucht S. Assessment of growth, part 2: interpretation of growth. Nutrition Focus 2000;15(3 and 4):1–16.
36. Adamkin DH. Pragmatic approach to in-hospital nutrition in high-risk neonates. J Perinatol 2005;25:S7–11.
37. Cooke R. Adjustable fortification of human milk fed to preterm infants. J Perinatol 2006;26(10):591–2.
38. Cooke RJ, Embleton N, Rigo J, et al. High protein pre-term infant formula: effect on nutrient balance metabolic status and growth. Pediatr Res 2006;59(2):265–70.
39. Heird WC. Biochemical homeostasis and body growth are reliable end points in clinical nutrition trials. Proc Nutr Soc 2005;64:297–303.
40. Gibson AT, Carney S, Cavazzoni E, et al. Neonatal and postnatal growth. Horm Res 2000;53(Suppl 1):42–9.
41. Sherry B, Mei Z, Grummer-Strawn L, et al. Evaluation of and recommendations for growth references for very low birth weight (<1500 grams) infants in the United States. Pediatrics 2003;111(4):750–8.
42. Hack M, Schluchter M, Cartar L, et al. Growth of very low birth weight infants to age 20 years. Pediatrics 2003;112:e30–8.
43. Lucas A. Early nutrition and later outcome. In: Ziegler EE, Lucas A, Moro GE, editors, Nutrition of the very low birthweight infant, vol. 43. Philadelphia: Nestec, Ltd., Vevey/Lippincott Williams & Wilkins; 1999. p. 1–18.
44. Foulder-Hughes LA, Cooke RWI. Motor, cognitive, and behavioural disorders in children born very preterm. Dev Med Child Neurol 2003;45(2):97–103.
45. Gale CR, O'Callaghan FJ, Bredow M, et al. The influence of head growth in fetal life, infancy, and childhood on the intelligence at the ages of 4 and 8 years. Pediatrics 2006;118:1486–92.
46. Latal-Hajnal B, von Siebenthal K, Kovari H, et al. Postnatal growth in VLBW infants: significant association with neurodevelopmental outcome. J Pediatr 2003;143(2):163–70.
47. Peterson J, Taylor HG, Minich N, et al. Subnormal head circumference in very low birth weight children: neonatal correlates and school-age consequences. Early Hum Dev 2006;82(5):325–34.
48. Babson S, Benda G. Growth graphs for the clinical assessment of infants of varying gestational age. Pediatrics 1976;89:814–20.
49. Uauy R, Tsang RC, Koletzko B, et al. Concepts, definitions and approaches to define the nutritional needs of LBW infants. In: Tsang RC, editor. Nutrition of the preterm infant: scientific basis and practical guidelines. 2nd edition. Cincinnati (OH): Digital Education al Publishing, Inc.; 2005.
50. Cockerill J, Uthaya S, Dore CJ, et al. Accelerated postnatal head growth follows preterm birth. Arch Dis Child Fetal Neonatal Ed 2006;91:F184–7.
51. Cooke RWI. Are there critical periods for brain growth in children born preterm? Arch Dis Child Fetal Neonatal Ed 2006;91:17–21.
52. Cooke RWI, Foulder-Hughes L. Growth impairment in the very preterm and cognitive and motor performance at 7 years. Arch Dis Child 2003;88:482–7.
53. Yeung M. Postnatal growth, neurodevelopment and altered adiposity after preterm birth from a clinical nutrition perspective. Acta Paediatr 2006;95:909–17.

54. Aggett PJ, Agostoni C, Axelsson I, et al. Feeding preterm infants after hospital discharge: a commentary by the ESPGHAN Committee on Nutrition. J Pediatr Gastroenterol Nutr 2006;42:596–603.
55. Gale CR, O'Callaghan FJ, Godfrey KM, et al. Critical periods of brain growth and cognitive function in children. Brain 2004;127:321–9.
56. Limperopoulos C, Soul JS, Gauvreau K, et al. Late gestation cerebellar growth is rapid and impeded by premature birth. Pediatrics 2005;115:688–95.
57. Hay WW. Early postnatal nutritional requirements of the very preterm infant based on a presentation at the NICHD-AAP Workshop on Research in Neonatology. J Perinatol 2006;26(S2):S13–8.
58. Cetin I, Alvino G, Radaelli T, et al. Fetal nutrition: a review. Acta Paediatr 2005;94:7–13.
59. Ibrahim HM, Jeroudi MA, Baier RJ, et al. Aggressive early total parental nutrition in low birth weight infants. J Perinatol 2004;24:482–6.
60. Farooqi A, Hagglof GS, Gotherfors L, et al. Growth in 10 to 12-year old children born at 23–25 weeks' gestation in the 1990s: a Swedish national prospective follow-up study. Pediatrics 2006;118:e1452–65.
61. Lainwala S, Perritt R, Poole KV, et al. Neurodevelopmental and growth outcomes of extremely low birth weight infants who are transferred from neonatal intensive care units to level I or II nurseries. Pediatrics 2007;119(5):e1079–87.
62. Aylward GP. Neurodevelopmental outcomes of infants born prematurely. J Dev Behav Pediatr 2005;26(6):427–37.
63. Davis NM, Ford GW, Anderson PJ, et al. Developmental coordination disorder at 8 years of age in a regional cohort of extremely low birthweight or very preterm infants. Dev Med Child Neurol 2007;49(5):325–30.
64. Adamkin DH. Nutrition management of the very low birthweight infant: optimizing enteral nutrition and post discharge nutrition. Neo Reviews 2006;7(12):216–21.
65. Koo WWK, Hockman EM. Posthospital discharge feeding for preterm infants: effects of standard compared with enriched milk formula on growth, bone mass, and body composition. Am J Clin Nutr 2006;84(6):1357–64.
66. Lucas A. Long-term programming effects of early nutrition—implications for the preterm infant. J Perinatol 2005;25:s2–6.
67. Zieglor EF, Lucas A, Moro GE. In: Nutrition of the very low birthweight infant, vol. 43. Philadelphia: Nestec, Ltd., Vevy/Lippincott Williams & Wilkins; 1999.
68. Barker DJP. The malnourished baby and infant: relationship with type 2 diabetes. Br Med Bull 2001;60(1):69–88.
69. Barker DJP. The origins of the developmental origins theory. J Intern Med 2007;261(5):412–7.
70. Van Aerde JE, Wilke MS, Feldman M, et al. Accretion of lipid in the fetus and newborn. In: Polin RA, Fox WW, Abman SH, editors, Fetal and neonatal physiology, vol. 1. 3rd edition. Philadelphia: Saunders; 2004. p. 388–404.
71. Kashyap S. Enteral intake for very low birth weight infants: what should the composition be? Semin Perinatol 2007;31:74–82.
72. Leitch C, Denne SC. Energy. In: Tsang RC, Uauy R, Koletzko B, et al, editors. Nutrition of the preterm infant. 2nd edition. Cincinnati (OH): Digital Educational Publishing, Inc.; 2005. p. 23–44.
73. Hay WW, Regnault TRH. Fetal requirements and placental transfer of nitrogenous compounds. In: Polin RA, Fox WW, Abman SH, editors, Fetal and neonatal physiology, vol. 1. 3rd edition. Philadelphia: Elsevier/Saunders; 2004. p. 509–27.

74. Kashyap S, Shultze KF, Forsyth M, et al. Growth, nutrient retention, and metabolic response in low birth weight infants fed varying intakes of protein and energy. J Pediatr 1988;113:713–21.
75. Kalhan SC, Iben S. Protein metabolism in the extremely low birth weight infant. Clin Perinatol 2000;27(1):23–55.
76. Hay WW. Intravenous nutrition of the very preterm neonate. Acta Paediatr 2005; 94(Suppl 449):47–56.
77. Berne RM, Levy MN, Koeppen BM, et al. Physiology. 5th edition. St. Louis: Mosby; 2004.
78. Heird WC, Kashyap S. Protein and amino acid metabolism and requirements. In: Polin RA, Fox WW, Abman SH, editors. Fetal and neonatal physiology, vol. 1. 3rd edition. Philadelphia: Saunders; 2004. p. 527–39.
79. Embleton N, Cooke RJ. Protein requirements in preterm infants: effect of different levels of protein intake on growth and body composition. Pediatr Res 2005;58(5): 855–60.
80. Michele JL, Fawer CL, Schutz Y. Protein requirement of the extremely low birthweight preterm infant. In: Ziegler EE, Lucas A, Moro GE, editors. Nutrition of the very low birthweight infant, vol. 43. Philadelphia: Nestec Ltd., Vevey/ Lippincott Williams & Wilkins; 1999. p. 155–78.
81. Olhager E, Forsum E. Total energy expenditure, body composition and weight gain in moderately preterm and full-term infants at term postconceptional age. Acta Paediatr 2003;92:1327–34.
82. te Braake FWJ, van den Akker CHP, Riedijk MA, et al. Parenteral amino acid and energy administration to premature infants in early life. Semin Fetal Neonatal Med 2007;12(1):11–8.
83. Yeung MY. Influence of early postnatal nutritional management on oxidative stress and antioxidant defense in extreme prematurity. Acta Paediatr 2006;95(2): 153–63.

# Congenital Adrenal Hyperplasia: An Endocrine Disorder with Neonatal Onset

Laura Stokowski, RN, MS

**KEYWORDS**

• Neonatal • Endocrine • Adrenal • Ambiguous genitalia
• Metabolic disorder • Salt-loss • Newborn • Genetic disorder

Our understanding of endocrine disorders in the neonate has increased in the wake of considerable advances in the fields of genetics and cell biology. In newborn nurseries and neonatal intensive care units (NICUs), endocrine dysfunction is encountered less often than disease of the respiratory, cardiac, or gastrointestinal system; in fact, we rarely think of it except when reviewing the results of a newborn metabolic screen. Endocrine dysfunction is deserving of our attention, however, because of the potentially grave consequences of unrecognized disease in the neonate. One acute clinical endocrine disorder manifesting shortly after birth is congenital adrenal hyperplasia (CAH), the most common cause of ambiguous genitalia in the newborn and, at times, the cause of sudden neonatal death. The management of a newborn with ambiguous genitalia has changed in recent years, and it is essential for caregivers to review the latest recommendations. The first part of this article reviews the pathophysiology and management of CAH, and the second deals with issues related to ambiguous genitalia in the CAH-affected child. To grasp the pathophysiology of CAH, a fundamental understanding of the endocrine system is required.

## THE ENDOCRINE SYSTEM

The classic endocrine system encompasses a diverse group of ductless secretory glands: the hypothalamus, pineal, pituitary, thyroid, parathyroid, thymus, pancreatic islet cells, adrenals, ovaries, and testes. Among the wide-ranging responsibilities of the endocrine system are coordination and regulation of metabolism, growth and development, and reproduction. The endocrine and central nervous systems are intimately linked, forming the neuroendocrine system, which has the complex task of controlling body homeostasis.

Neonatal Intensive Care Unit, Inova Fairfax Hospital for Children, 3300 Gallows Road, Falls Church, VA 22042, USA
*E-mail address:* stokowski@cox.net

Crit Care Nurs Clin N Am 21 (2009) 195–212
doi:10.1016/j.ccell.2009.01.008 **ccnursing.theclinics.com**
0899-5885/09/$ – see front matter 

Endocrine glands and tissues throughout the body synthesize, store, and secrete hormones, the chemical messengers of the neuroendocrine system. After secretion into the blood or extracellular fluid, hormones exert their actions on specific target cells located in nearby or distant tissues. Target cells contain specific receptors to which corresponding hormones must attach to exert physiologic actions.

Hormones are powerful negative feedback regulators of their own production. As hormones reach target levels, the anterior pituitary and hypothalamus are suppressed, ceasing production of the respective trophic and releasing hormones. Endocrine disease can be associated with hormone overproduction, hormone underproduction, or altered tissue responses to hormones.[1] The endocrine disorder CAH involves a failure to produce the hormones cortisol and aldosterone, along with inappropriate production of androgens.

### *Adrenal Hormones*

The adrenal glands are located at the superior poles of the kidneys. Each gland is composed of two distinct independently functioning organs: the inner medulla, which produces catecholamines, and the outer cortex, which synthesizes three classes of steroid hormones (mineralocorticoids, glucocorticoids, and androgens). Adrenal steroid production and regulation require a functional hypothalamic-pituitary-adrenal (HPA) axis.

The release of cortisol, the body's major glucocorticoid, is controlled by regulating its rate of synthesis. Central nervous stimulation, such as that associated with stress, surgery, extreme heat or cold, hypoxia, infection, hypoglycemia, or injury, prompts the release of corticotropin-releasing factor (CRF) from the hypothalamus. CRF binds to receptors in the anterior pituitary, where it stimulates the release of corticotropin into the bloodstream. In the adrenal cortex, corticotropin stimulates the synthesis and release of cortisol. The increasing circulating cortisol level exerts negative feedback stimulation on the hypothalamus and anterior pituitary to suppress CRF and corticotropin, respectively, thereby inhibiting further production of cortisol. This regulatory system is known as a closed negative feedback loop (**Fig. 1**).

Aldosterone, the chief mineralocorticoid, regulates the renal retention of sodium and water and the excretion of potassium. Aldosterone is critical to electrolyte balance, blood pressure, and intravascular volume and is itself regulated by the plasma renin-angiotensin (PRA) system. Renin, released by the kidneys, stimulates the formation of angiotensin, a powerful vasoconstrictor that, in turn, stimulates the release of aldosterone from the adrenal cortex.

The adrenal androgens (dehydroepiandrosterone [DHEA], DHEA sulfate, and androstenedione) are regulated by corticotropin. These steroids have minimal androgenic activity on their own but are converted in the peripheral tissues to two more potent androgens, testosterone and dihydrotestosterone (DHT). These latter hormones are largely responsible for virilization of the external genitalia in the male fetus.

## CONGENITAL ADRENAL HYPERPLASIA

CAH is a deficiency in one of five enzymes required to synthesize cortisol from cholesterol in the adrenal cortex. Mutations in the 21-hydroxylase (21-OHD) gene, of which there are more than 50, are, by a large margin, the most frequent cause of CAH.[2] The 21-OHD form of CAH accounts for 95% of cases and is the chief cause of ambiguous genitalia in the neonate. Of the remaining four relatively rare enzyme deficiencies, 11β-hydroxylase deficiency is most frequent. A recently described type of CAH is P450

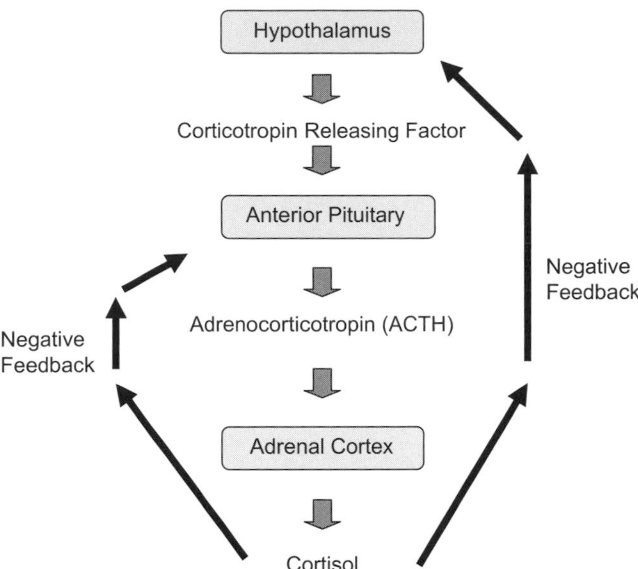


**Fig. 1.** HPA axis control of cortisol. Hypothalamic corticotropin-releasing factor (CRF) stimulates the anterior pituitary to produce corticotropin, which stimulates the adrenal cortex to produce cortisol. The increasing cortisol level exerts negative feedback stimulation on the anterior pituitary and hypothalamus to stop releasing CRF and corticotropin.

oxidoreductase (POR) deficiency, an autosomal recessive disorder of steroidogenesis that involves partial deficiencies of 21-OHD, 17$\alpha$-hydroxylase, and 17/20-lyase enzymes and is associated with skeletal malformations.[3]

Classic 21-OHD CAH is not a single disease but a continuum of enzyme impairment from minimal to absolute, producing corresponding clinical manifestations ranging from a simple virilizing form of CAH to severe salt-wasting disease.[4] 21-OHD deficiency occurs in approximately 1 in 15,000 live births, although pockets of increased incidence are found in a few areas around the world. A milder nonclassic form is much more common but is rarely detected before adolescence.[4]

## *Pathophysiology*

Partial activity or complete absence of the 21-OHD enzyme disrupts the process of adrenosteroid synthesis (**Fig. 2**). In the first two steps of the normal steroidogenic pathway, cholesterol is converted to progesterone and then to two end products, aldosterone and cortisol. In 21-OHD deficiency, both of these pathways are blocked, preventing the synthesis of aldosterone and cortisol. The decreasing cortisol level stimulates the pituitary to secrete corticotropin in a vain attempt to generate more cortisol. The chronically stimulated fetal adrenal cortex enlarges, becoming the characteristic anatomic feature from which the disorder takes its name.[4] The obstructed steroid pathway also produces an accumulation of precursors, particularly 17-hydroxyprogesterone (17-OHP), upstream of the blocked step. Surplus 17-OHP is diverted into the unobstructed androgen pathway, becoming the substrate for the synthesis of adrenal androgen precursors that are converted to testosterone in peripheral tissues.[5]

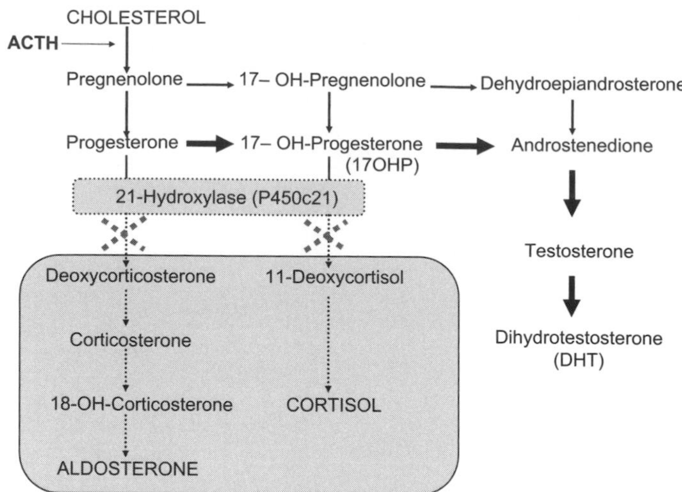


**Fig. 2.** Pathophysiology of 21-hydroxylase (21-OHD) deficiency. The steroidogenic pathway represents the pathophysiology of 21-OHD deficiency. A deficiency of 21-OHD prevents conversion of cholesterol to cortisol and aldosterone. Precursors, including 17-hydroxyprogesterone (17-OHP), proximal to the blocked step are shunted into the androgen synthesis pathway, resulting in an excess of androgens. (*From* Kenner C, Lott J. Comprehensive neonatal care. 4th edition. Philadelphia: Saunders Elsevier; 2007. p. 163; with permission.)

Hence, the main consequence of blocked cortisol and aldosterone production is an excess of circulating sex steroids. At critical periods in fetal development, these inappropriate yet potent androgens (testosterone and its active metabolite, DHT) bind to receptors in the fetal external genitalia, inducing them to develop in a male fashion. This process is known as virilization or masculinization of the external genitalia. The excess testosterone has little effect, if any, on the male (XY) fetus, but in the female (XX) fetus, these androgens masculinize the genitalia to varying degrees.[5] Internal reproductive organs (ovaries, fallopian tubes, and uterus) are not affected by this degree of androgen exposure and develop normally. Without treatment, virilization of the child is progressive, culminating in precocious puberty, advanced bone age, and other problems.[4] Cortisol is also required for the conversion of norepinephrine to epinephrine in the adrenal medulla; thus, the infant with CAH also has a low epinephrine level.[5]

## *Clinical Manifestations*

The clinical and biochemical features of classic 21-OHD CAH arise from the hormonal imbalances just described.[6] Because so many gene mutations are associated with CAH, a broad array of clinical manifestations is possible.[5] Approximately three fourths of affected infants have a concurrent aldosterone deficiency; these infants are known as "salt-losers" or "salt-wasters" because of their propensity to excrete excessive amounts of sodium in the urine. The salt-losing state is delayed until the postnatal period, because fetal fluid and electrolyte balance is regulated by the placenta and maternal kidneys.[5] Salt loss, which generally develops in the second week of life, can have an earlier onset.

In addition to urinary sodium loss, the urinary excretion of potassium is not efficient in the infant who has CAH.[6] Glucose homeostasis is problematic as well because of the role of cortisol in stimulating the release of glucose. If uncorrected, these derangements can lead to profound and life-threatening hyponatremia, hyperkalemia, hypovolemia, hypoglycemia, and dehydration.

The remaining 25% of infants with classic 21-OHD have an incomplete enzymatic block and are able to synthesize enough aldosterone to maintain fluid and electrolyte homeostasis. This form is known as "simple virilizing CAH," because the chief clinical finding is the effect of androgen excess on the external genitalia.

Girls affected by 21-OHD deficiency are usually recognized at birth by their atypical genitals. Variable assessment findings include clitoromegaly, posterior fusion of the labia majora, and a single perineal orifice instead of separate urethral and vaginal openings.[7] In the latter finding, the vagina joins the urethra above the perineum, forming a urogenital sinus. In the most severe cases, a urethra is enclosed within the phallus and the girl is mistaken for a boy with bilateral cryptorchidism and hypospadias (**Fig. 3**).[8] Hyperpigmentation of the genital skin is a consequence of excessive pituitary corticotropin secretion. Male infants with 21-OHD appear normal or, at most, have enlarged genitals. The disease may not be detected in male newborns during the immediate neonatal period, because the onset of adrenal symptoms is delayed until 5 to 14 days of life. Undiagnosed infants may present to the emergency room with signs and symptoms of impending adrenal collapse: vomiting, weight loss, lethargy, severe dehydration, electrolyte imbalances, hypoglycemia, hypovolemia, shock, and a normal anion gap acidosis.[9]

### *Diagnosis*

Measurement of serum 17-OHP concentration is the principal means of confirming the diagnosis of CAH. Samples should be drawn in the early morning before 8:00 AM.[8] A markedly elevated 17-OHP level suggests classic 21-OHD deficiency. Random 17-OHP levels in affected newborns can reach 10,000 ng/dL (normal is <100 ng/dL).[8] These extremely high basal 17-OHP levels may not be reached until the second or third day of life; thus, the results of a specimen drawn in the first 24 hours could lead to false assurance that the newborn does not have CAH. Repeated testing 24 hours later may be required to demonstrate an elevation in 17-OHP level.[8] If the 17-OHP increase is only mild to moderate, a 60-minute corticotropin test provides

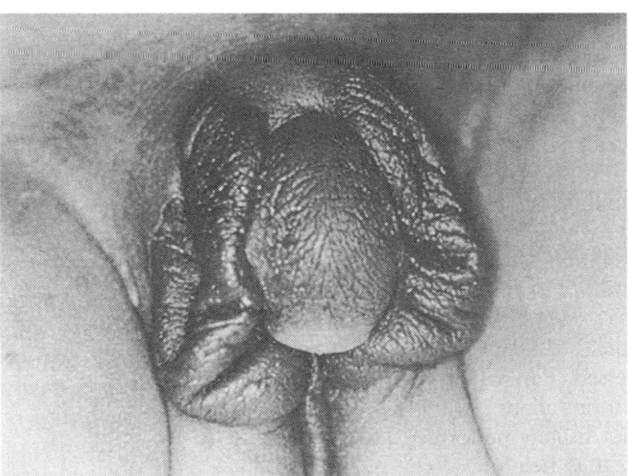

**Fig. 3.** External genitalia of a 46XX neonate who has CAH. Features include clitoromegaly and rugosed, hyperpigmented, and partly fused labioscrotal folds. (*From* Kenner C, Lott J. Comprehensive neonatal care, 4th edition. Philadelphia: Saunders Elsevier 2007; p. 163; with permission.)

a more reliable diagnosis.[10] In neonates who have CAH, 17-OHP increases in response to exogenous corticotropin administration but cortisol does not.

Biochemical support for the diagnosis of CAH also includes elevated serum DHEA and androstenedione levels in male and female babies, and elevated serum testosterone in female babies. Infants with salt-losing disease often have serum sodium levels less than 110 mEq/L and serum potassium levels as high as 10 mEq/L.[5] Serum pH may be less than 7.1, with hypotension and shock that are fatal if untreated. Hypoglycemia may be present as well. Molecular genetic analysis is not usually essential for the diagnosis but may be helpful to confirm the exact type of defect and to aid in determining recurrence risk for CAH in future siblings. A karyotype or fluorescence in situ hybridization test for sex chromosome material is needed when ambiguous genitalia are encountered or the suspected diagnosis is CAH. Some infants are so externally virilized that it might be difficult for parents to believe the infant is genetically female without the proof presented by chromosome testing.

Imaging studies, such as pelvic and abdominal ultrasound, reveal a uterus (if present), assess adrenal size, and more rapidly identify the gender of the infant. Although fallopian tubes and ovaries are not always visible on ultrasound, it is usually possible to identify the uterus.[11] Endoscopic and fluoroscopic studies are further options to define internal anatomy.

### *Newborn Screening for Congenital Adrenal Hyperplasia*

Occasionally, a newborn who has CAH is born without genital ambiguity and demonstrates no early clinical signs or symptoms of glucocorticoid or mineralocorticoid deficiency. These infants remain undiagnosed, and without treatment, they are at risk for life-threatening salt-losing crisis.[6] This is the rationale for neonatal screening for CAH, conducted at the same time as mandatory screening for hypothyroidism, phenylketonuria, and other genetic disorders.

The increased serum 17-OHP levels in affected neonates permit screening for the disorder using blood filter specimens. As of 2008, all 50 states mandate newborn screening for CAH,[12] the objectives of which are the presymptomatic identification of neonates at risk for adrenal crisis and prevention of incorrect gender assignment of affected female newborns with ambiguous genitalia. False-positive results can occur in preterm newborns or sick newborns, both of whom typically have higher levels of 17-OHP. A 4:1 preponderance of CAH in female neonates compared with male neonates in countries without neonatal screening for CAH suggests that boys are dying in infancy before a diagnosis of CAH is made.[13] Neonatal screening can also detect a portion of babies with nonclassic CAH.

### *Management*

Because urgent medical attention can be lifesaving for the newborn who has CAH, physiologic replacement dosing of glucocorticoid is begun as soon as the diagnosis is confirmed. The goal of therapy is to prevent corticotropin and androgen overproduction, without completely suppressing the HPA axis.[14] Aldosterone replacement maintains fluid and electrolyte homeostasis, and dietary sodium supplementation is often necessary. Agents of choice for treatment in the newborn are hydrocortisone (a glucocorticoid) plus fludrocortisone (a mineralocorticoid). Further clinical management is guided by daily weights, serum adrenal steroid concentrations, PRA, electrolytes, blood glucose, and other data. Plasma renin activity should be compared with age-specific norms, because basal PRA is higher in the newborn than in older infants. Children with classic 21-OHD are unable to produce sufficient cortisol in response to physiologic stress, such as fever, surgery, or trauma. These patients need increased hydrocortisone (stress dosing) during such times.[4]

### *Gender Issues*

Although most genetic female newborns who have CAH eventually develop a female gender identity, this outcome can be unpredictable.[8,15] In some populations, some significantly virilized XX children raised as female reverted at various ages to male sexual identities.[15] Male-like behaviors, abilities, and identities in CAH-affected female children are thought to be a consequence of hormonal imprinting of the brain in the developing fetus.[8] It is acknowledged that there is insufficient understanding of the impact of prenatal androgen exposure on the fetal central nervous system and how this exposure affects future development.[16] There is evidence that fetal androgen exposure influences gender identity and role behavior, but the extent and timing of requisite exposure are unknown.[17,18] Given the likelihood of identifying with the female gender, in addition to their potential fertility, it is generally recommended that genetic newborns who have CAH be raised as girls, even when initially misassigned as boys.[19] Some parents do elect to raise their overtly virilized genetically female newborns as boys, however, particularly when there is a delayed diagnosis.[20]

Parents are understandably concerned and anxious about the appearance of the external genitalia in their virilized female newborns. For most, ambiguous genitalia are outside the sphere of their knowledge and experience, and they have many questions about the significance, permanence, or possible treatment of their child's condition. Hypertrophy of the clitoris may gradually abate with medical therapy, but severe virilization does not spontaneously reverse. The option of genital surgery is usually delayed until the infant is 2 to 6 months of age. It may be helpful for the parents to meet with the pediatric urologic surgeon during the initial hospitalization or shortly afterward to allay their anxiety and begin to become informed about the options that require their thoughtful consideration. One alternative is to delay cosmetic surgery for mild to moderate clitoromegaly until the child is old enough to participate in the decision;[19] another is to omit surgery altogether for infants with milder virilization.[16] When surgery is necessary for the female child with CAH, the goals are to achieve unobstructed urinary emptying without incontinence or infections and good adult sexual and reproductive function. Such procedures should be undertaken only by experienced surgeons who use techniques that avoid disrupting the neurovascular complex supplying the clitoris.[16] Functional outcome of the genitalia should take precedence over appearance.[16]

### *Discharge Planning*

CAH is not limited to the newborn period; it is a permanent disorder that presents management challenges throughout the individual's lifetime.[5] After discharge, infants who have CAH must be closely followed by a pediatric endocrinologist for assessments of hormone levels, blood sugar, blood pressure, growth, maturity, skeletal maturation, and other parameters necessary to guard against over- or undertreatment. The parents must be educated about the importance of adhering to the prescribed medical therapy and keeping all medical appointments for clinical and laboratory monitoring.[5] Parents should be advised that early rapid growth of the child may necessitate frequent dosage adjustment of replacement hormones and that higher dosing of medications is required in times of physiologic stress.[5] The parents should also be referred to a geneticist for counseling regarding future pregnancies. Prenatal diagnosis and treatment of CAH are possible, if still controversial. Started early enough in the pregnancy, dexamethasone given to the mother can minimize or eliminate virilization of female offspring.[21]

## AMBIGUOUS GENITALIA

Developmental deviations of the external genitalia requiring further investigation occur in approximately 1 in 4000 newborns.[22] The currently accepted term for a disorder that alters genital development is *disorder of sex development* (DSD), a congenital condition in which development of the chromosomal, gonadal, or anatomic gender is atypical.[23] In CAH, only the anatomic gender is affected. The question in the minds of parents, expressed or not, is how can a baby girl be born looking like a baby boy? To answer this, one must consider the bipotential nature of human sexual development and how genes and hormones interact to guide this development.

### *Sexual Differentiation of the Fetus*

During the early weeks of development, all embryos have undifferentiated gonads capable of becoming testes or ovaries. This first developmental stage is dictated by genes. Male-specific development requires the expression of the testis-determining gene (SRY) located on the short arm of the Y-chromosome, which stimulates differentiation of the gonads to testes. If the Y-chromosome is absent, the gonads become ovaries.

Subsequent events in sexual development are hormonally mediated. By 7 weeks of gestation, each fetus has two sets of primitive ducts, the müllerian (female) and the wolffian (male), only one of which is retained to become the internal reproductive organs. Further, in male fetuses, the testes develop two types of hormone-producing cells: the Sertoli cells and the Leydig cells. The Sertoli cells begin secreting müllerian inhibiting factor (MIF), which causes the müllerian ducts to regress. The testicular Leydig cells secrete the androgens necessary for further masculinization of the fetus. Testosterone acts locally in high concentrations to induce maturation of the wolffian ducts into the epididymis, vas deferens, and seminal vesicles of the male fetus.

The female fetus does not produce MIF or testicular testosterone; thus, the wolffian ducts regress. The müllerian ducts, which do not require ovarian hormones for further development, become the fallopian tubes, uterus, and upper vagina.

Lastly, the budding external genital structures of male and female fetuses are identical. In both genders, this primitive stage is characterized by formation of a genital tubercle that elongates to form a phallus and a urogenital sinus that is surrounded by inner urogenital folds and outer labioscrotal swellings (**Fig. 4**). Between the eighth and 14th weeks of gestation, the fetal hormonal milieu dictates the course that further development takes. If the fetus produces DHT, this potent metabolite of testosterone binds to androgen receptors in the genital tissues and induces male-typical development: the urethral folds fuse to form the penile shaft, the labioscrotal swellings evolve into the scrota, and the urogenital sinus becomes the male urethra.

In the absence of DHT, the external genitalia develop in a female fashion. The genital tubercle becomes a clitoris, and the labioscrotal swellings remain unfused to form the labia majora and minora. The urogenital sinus develops into the lower vagina and urethra. Feminine external genital development is complete by 11 weeks of gestation. At this juncture, however, the altered steroid biosynthesis of 21-OHD CAH disrupts the finely orchestrated development of the fetal genitalia.

In the first trimester, placental aromatase is not yet sufficient to convert androgens to estrogens and to protect the female external genitalia from the effects of testosterone.[24] The testosterone produced by the adrenal cortex as a consequence of blocked cortisol production is free to act on the genital tissues of the female fetus in the same way it does in the male fetus, inducing growth of the clitoris, fusion of the labioscrotal folds, and failure of the urogenital sinus to become a lower vagina.

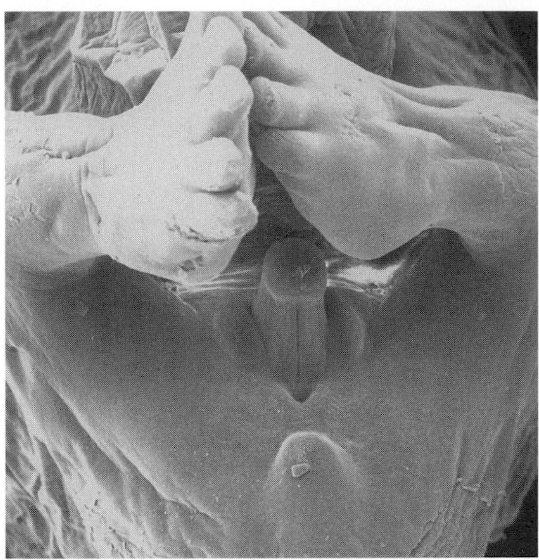

**Fig. 4.** Fetal external genitalia at approximately 53 days after fertilization, demonstrating the lack of differentiation in the external genitalia at this stage of development. (*Courtesy of* K. Sulik, PhD, Chapel Hill, NC.)

Testosterone exposure at this sensitive stage can even produce a penile urethra and prevent the vagina from fully descending into the perineum, leaving a urogenital canal that ends in a blind pouch. Testosterone exposure beyond this point can increase growth of the clitoris but does not fuse the labia or create a penile urethra.[25]

## *Disorders of Sex Development*

Although the most common DSD in the neonate is CAH, there are other conditions that result in ambiguous genitalia. Possible, yet rare, causes of virilization of external genitalia in the 46XX newborn include placental aromatase deficiency, maternal androgen-producing or adrenal tumors, and medications with androgenic action taken during the first trimester of pregnancy. In the newborn whose karyotype is not yet known, and in whom no syndrome is evident, other possible etiologies of ambiguous genitalia are mixed gonadal dysgenesis, partial androgen insensitivity syndrome (PAIS), and testosterone biosynthetic defects. Newborns affected by cloacal exstrophy also exhibit disruption of genital development but are immediately identified by their pelvic anomalies.

### *Clinical assessment*

A complete evaluation of the neonate with genital ambiguity requires a detailed family history. History that suggests CAH includes consanguinity, genital ambiguity in other family members, or a previous neonatal death, possibly from an undiagnosed adrenal crisis. Virilizing changes in the mother that reverse after delivery suggest aromatase deficiency.[23]

A detailed examination of the genitalia must be conducted. The first and all subsequent examinations should respect the privacy of the child and the family as much as possible, avoiding overexposure of the infant even for educational purposes.[26] Although physical assessment alone does not permit a firm diagnosis of CAH or other DSD, some assessment findings can guide the diagnostic process in one direction or another. A precise description of the anatomy is most useful for documenting this assessment, but the examiner may wish to assess the degree of virilization using Prader staging. A female newborn with mild clitoromegaly is classified as Prader stage II, and stage V represents a typical male newborn (**Fig. 5**). The examiner should look for symmetry or asymmetry of the genitalia. In the virilized female neonate, genitalia are symmetric, whereas in other DSDs, asymmetry of labia or scrota may be apparent. Experienced examiners may be able to palpate a uterus by digital rectal examination as an anterior midline cordlike structure.

The examiner should palpate for testes in the scrota or inguinal canal, which is possibly the most important finding in terms of establishing gender.[27] A palpable testis excludes the diagnosis of a virilized genetic female (46XX) newborn who has CAH. A unilateral testis points to an undescended testis or a different DSD, such as mixed gonadal dysgenesis or ovotesticular DSD.[27] To locate testes, the examiner's finger is placed flat and moved down along the line of the inguinal canal on each side, beginning well above the site of the internal inguinal ring.

Clitoral size should be measured if clitoromegaly is present. Clitoral length greater than 1 cm in term newborns is considered excessive. Clitoral size often seems large in preterm newborns, because clitoral breadth is the same at 27 weeks as it is at term. A prominent but not truly enlarged clitoris is a normal assessment finding that often prompts referrals for genital ambiguity.[28]

The examiner next assesses the labioscrotal folds. Labial fullness, a benign finding, is another feature occasionally mistaken for genital ambiguity. The labioscrotal folds are examined for fusion, which starts posteriorly and moves anteriorly, increasing the anogenital distance.[7] The perineum is inspected by gently separating the labia and using an examination light to confirm the presence of separate urethral and vaginal openings or a single urogenital orifice (an opening connected to urinary and genital systems).[7] Note rugosity or hyperpigmentation of labioscrotal folds, signifying hypersecretion of corticotropin associated with CAH.

### *Further Investigations*

DSDs are diagnosed with a combination of biochemical, hormonal, and genetic testing. The principal aim of an initial investigation is to rule out a life-threatening illness, such as CAH, which can precipitate an adrenal crisis (see previous section for typical diagnostic studies for CAH). Other investigations, such as serum MIF, luteinizing hormone (LH), follicle-stimulating hormone, human chorionic gonadotropin (hCG) stimulation test, or urinary steroid analysis, may be undertaken if the examination suggests that the newborn is not a virilized genetic girl but has a different DSD or a different (rarer) type of CAH. The hCG stimulation test, performed after 24 hours of

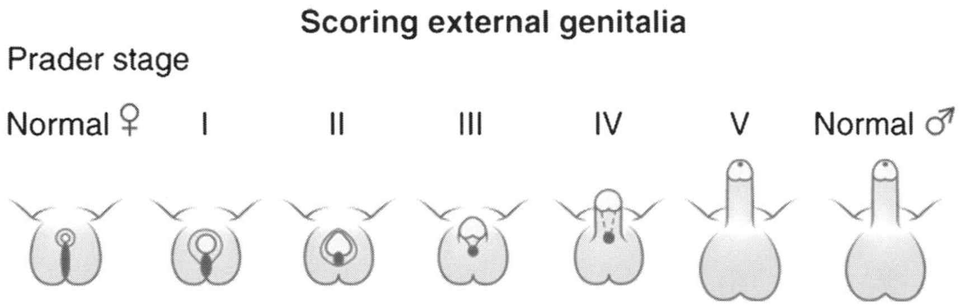

**Fig. 5.** Prader staging tool for evaluation of genital virilization. (*From* Kenner C, Lott J. Comprehensive neonatal care, 4th edition. Philadelphia: Saunders Elsevier 2007; p. 168; with permission.)

life, essentially evaluates the newborn's ability to produce age-appropriate androgen concentrations.[29] Molecular genetic analysis may be required to provide a definitive diagnosis for some disorders.

In the most recent consensus of experts, DSDs are classified according to karyotype (**Box 1**).[23] Provisional diagnostic groupings, based on the presence or absence of a uterus, symmetry of the external genitalia, and presence of gonads, provide a basis for more focused additional investigation of the infant with genital ambiguity (**Table 1**).[30] In addition to 21-OHD deficiency, more common causes of ambiguous genitalia include gonadal dysgenesis, PAIS, and testosterone biosynthetic defects.

## BIRTH OF CHILD WITH A DISORDER OF SEX DEVELOPMENT

Failure to assign a definitive gender at the time of birth is extremely distressing to families.[29] Parents of children born with a DSD report many instances of overreaction, drama, and unnecessary panic on the part of health care professionals in the delivery room.[26] On birth of a child with atypical genitalia, labor and delivery personnel must behave in a calm and thoughtful manner.[26] Naive or insensitive comments regarding the baby in the immediate hours after birth can become imprinted in the parents' minds.[26,29] Inappropriate terms, information overload, or contradictory information can cause misunderstandings and psychologic harm that outlasts the hospitalization.[26,29] The number of people directly involved with the parents should be minimized to avoid overwhelming them.[26] This is particularly important in teaching institutions, where it may be tempting to use the newborn as a teaching opportunity. Health care personnel should maintain an environment of dignity and privacy, whether during an examination of the baby or a discussion with the parents. Confidentiality is of the utmost importance.[26] If conditions allow, the baby should be permitted to remain with the mother for bonding. Sending a baby unnecessarily to the NICU interferes with bonding between parent and child and, unless a private room is available, exposes the parents to questions from curious visitors about the baby's gender or reason for admission.

### *Talking with Families*

Optimal care of the child who has a DSD involves a patient-centered approach.[26] Many centers manage the care of these newborns with a well-coordinated multidisciplinary team.[11] Team members may include the attending neonatologist, neonatal nurse, endocrinologist, pediatric surgeon or pediatric urologic surgeon, social worker, counselor or other mental health professional, and, in some instances, geneticist. The role of the nurse on the multidisciplinary team is to coordinate routine care of the baby, provide practical instruction and support to the parents, reinforce education and management principles, and connect families with resources and support services. The nurse also communicates parental concerns and questions back to the team.[26] Nurse practitioners on the team often function as team coordinator or team liaison between the team and the family.[26]

A single individual should be identified to communicate diagnostic findings and plans to the family. When discussing possible diagnoses with the family, language must be carefully chosen. The terms *hermaphrodite*, *pseudohermaphrodite*, and *intersex* are outdated, confusing, and perceived as distasteful by many.[16] These words should be avoided; instead, accurate informative terms that describe the baby's diagnosis should be used. A clear explanation of sexual development in the fetus can help parents to understand how development of their newborn deviated from normal, which is an important prerequisite for parental coping.[28] When conveying

**Box 1**
**Disorders associated with ambiguous genitalia**

*Sex chromosome DSD*

- 45,X Turner syndrome
- 45,X/46,XY gonadal dysgenesis
- 46,XX/46,XY gonadal dysgenesis

*46,XY DSD*

Disorders of testicular development

- Complete or partial gonadal dysgenesis
- Ovotesticular DSD
- Testes regression

Disorders of androgen synthesis

- 5α-reductase 2 deficiency
- LH receptor mutations
- Steroidogenic acute regulatory protein mutation
- Cholesterol side-chain cleavage mutation
- 3β-hydroxysteroid dehydrogenase 2 deficiency
- 17β-hydroxysteroid dehydrogenase deficiency
- 17α-hydroxylase/17,20-lyase deficiency
- POR deficiency

Disorders of androgen action

- Androgen insensitivity syndrome
- Environmental or drug effects

Other

- Syndromes (eg, cloacal anomalies)
- Persistent müllerian duct syndrome
- Vanishing testes syndrome
- Isolated hypospadias
- Congenital hypogonadotropic hypogonadism
- Cryptorchidism
- Environmental influences

*46,XX DSD*

Disorders of ovarian development

- Gonadal dysgenesis
- Ovotesticular DSD
- Testicular DSD

Disorders of androgen excess

- Fetal
    - 21-OHD deficiency
    - 3β-hydroxysteroid dehydrogenase 2 deficiency

  - POR deficiency
  - 11β-hydroxylase deficiency
  - Glucocorticoid receptor mutations
- Fetoplacental
  - Aromatase deficiency
  - Oxidoreductase deficiency
- Maternal
  - Maternal virilizing tumor
  - Androgenic drugs

Other

- Syndromes (eg, cloacal anomalies)
- Müllerian agenesis
- Uterine anomalies
- Vaginal atresia

*Adapted from* Hughes IA. Disorders of sex development: a new definition and classification. Best Pract Res Clin Endocrinol Metab 2008;22:122; with permission.

the results of tests to parents, it is important to pair this with an explanation of the significance of those tests. Problems arise when health professionals themselves have misunderstandings regarding test results. A good example of this is the significance of karyotype results. Having a Y-chromosome does not make an individual male, because much more than the Y-chromosome is required for male development, such as the ability of cells to respond to androgens.[26] Nor does the lack of a Y-chromosome make a person female. A Y-chromosome can be translocated onto an X-chromosome; thus, an individual with a 46XX karyotype can develop along male lines.[26] It can facilitate parents' understanding and acceptance if they are aware that a person's genes alone do not determine gender.

**Table 1**
**Diagnostic groupings of disorders of sex development based on initial examination**

| Findings | Disorder(s) Suggested |
|---|---|
| Uterus<br>No palpable gonads<br>Symmetric external genitalia<br>Hyperpigmentation | CAH (21-OHD) in virilized female infant |
| Uterus<br>Palpable gonads<br>Asymmetric external genitalia | Gonadal dysgenesis with Y-chromosome or true gonadal dysgenesis |
| No uterus<br>Palpable gonads<br>Symmetric external genitalia | Undervirilized XY male infant (PAIS or testosterone biosynthetic defect) |

*From* Kenner C, Lott JW. Comprehensive neonatal care. 4th edition. Philadelphia: Saunders Elsevier, 2007; with permission.

It is the parents who have the ultimate responsibility to make or defer decisions about care for their child who has a DSD, including gender of rearing and surgery.[28] The role of the health care team is to provide information, share and explain all diagnostic findings, inform the parents of all available options, and support the parents in the decision-making process. Support for parental uncertainty must also be provided. The approach must also be culturally sensitive. Communication should be open and honest, including candid discussion of the controversies and dilemmas concerning gender assignment and early genital surgery.

The parents of a child who has a DSD need psychosocial support. Psychologic evaluation should include an assessment of the parents' expectations regarding the gender of their baby, their understanding of what they have been told since the baby's birth, their coping mechanisms, and their preferences for care and treatment of the baby.[11] Parental acceptance of the child who has a DSD is a key determinant of a favorable outcome.[28]

### *Gender Assignment*

Parents are naturally anxious to find out their baby's gender so that they can name the baby and announce the birth to family and friends. Nevertheless, it must be sensitively communicated that although their distress is acknowledged, when gender is in doubt, a gender-of-rearing decision is one with lifelong implications and cannot be made in haste. A key element in gender-of-rearing decisions is the gender that the child is most likely to identify with when older.[26] Although 90% of children who have CAH, and 100% of those affected with complete androgen insensitivity syndrome, continue to identify with the female gender, the concordance between gender of rearing and gender identity is less clearcut in other DSDs. In disorders that involve virilization at puberty, such as 5-α-reductase deficiency, there is a significant likelihood of the individual identifying as male at that time.[29]

Gender assignment must be deferred until sufficient data are available for a fully informed decision. Unfortunately, some tests required for evaluation of DSDs must be sent out to referral laboratories, and the long wait for results can be frustrating for the parents. Parents wonder what to tell family and friends about the baby. It is helpful if an experienced mental health professional can meet early with the parents to help them formulate what to tell family and friends while awaiting a diagnosis.[31] Although it may feel awkward, parents should be open and honest with others regarding the child's condition. Instead of withholding information or lying, this approach lessens any shame and embarrassment that parents may feel.[26]

Surgery for a DSD is rarely performed in the neonatal period.[26] An exception is the neonate who requires the surgical creation of a urinary opening. In the past, early cosmetic surgery was frequently performed to reduce parental anxiety and make the child look "normal." In lieu of the rush to surgery, a more cautious approach to childhood cosmetic surgery is gaining acceptance. It is now preferable to avoid surgery in infancy and childhood and to preserve the integrity of genital tissue.[23]

The following case study illustrates the key elements of care for the child and family after the birth of a newborn with CAH.

## CASE STUDY

A baby was born by spontaneous vaginal delivery at 40 weeks of gestation after an uncomplicated pregnancy. Apgar scores were 8 and 9. In the delivery room, the obstetrician announced that the newborn was a boy, confirming what the parents had been expecting, because a second-trimester sonogram had identified the gender of the fetus as male.

While conducting the newborn physical examination a short time later, the nurse noted that no testes were palpable and the baby had hypospadias. She notified the pediatrician, who examined the baby and informed the parents that it was now not certain that the baby was a boy and that more tests needed to be done.

### *Physical Assessment and History*

A more detailed examination revealed that the newborn's "scrota" were symmetric and rugose but empty. No testes were palpable in the scrotal sacs or in the inguinal canals. The scrotal folds were fused in the midline. The phallus measured 2 cm. A single urogenital opening was found on the perineum, at the base of the phallus, from which the neonate was seen to void. The newborn did not have any dysmorphic features. A history obtained from the parents was negative for similarly affected infants or other relatives, neonatal death, maternal virilization, or consanguinity. The neonate was clinically stable, with normal vital signs, blood pressure, and blood glucose.

### *Diagnosis*

Based on the absence of palpable gonads, the most likely diagnosis was female virilization. A virilized female baby can look much like an undervirilized male baby, however, so it was important to confirm that no testes were present before assigning gender. In the meantime, the differential diagnosis included all the various causes of male undervirilization (PAIS, 5-$\alpha$-reductase deficiency, and testosterone biosynthetic defects). Because the genitalia were symmetric in appearance, mixed gonadal dysgenesis and true gonadal DSD were considered unlikely.

Initial investigations for this newborn included peripheral blood karyotype, 17-OHP, DHEA, progesterone, testosterone, androstenedione, cortisol, plasma renin activity, and electrolytes. A pelvic/abdominal ultrasound was ordered, and a pediatric endocrinology consult was initiated.

Many of the tests for evaluation of hormonal deficiencies and genetic disorders must be sent to specialized laboratories, and the results take days or even weeks. In this case, a working diagnosis was formulated based on the early hormonal and chemistry results and the results of the pelvic/abdominal ultrasound. The serum 17-OHP was 168 nmol/L on day 1 and 437 nmol/L on day 2. DHEA, progesterone, testosterone, and androstenedione were all elevated. Cortisol was low. Serum electrolytes were normal.

These results are consistent with a diagnosis of CAH caused by 21-OHD deficiency. Although the 17-OHP was only mildly elevated on day 1, the 17-OHP level increased further on day 2. The other steroid levels supported this diagnosis. The pelvic ultrasound revealed enlarged adrenal glands and a normal uterus; no testes were visualized. Karyotype results take longer, but the ultrasound confirmed that the baby was a genetic (46XX) female.

### *Management*

Treatment for 21-OHD deficiency was initiated immediately to prevent the onset of salt-wasting. The pediatric endocrinologist was identified as the person who would communicate diagnostic findings and treatment plans to the family.

While awaiting test results, the newborn stayed with her mother in a private room. Feedings were well tolerated, and the newborn remained clinically and biochemically stable. Even though, in most cases, the signs of adrenal insufficiency are not apparent until after the first week, in rare cases, it can begin earlier. The pediatric endocrinologist met with the family and explained the diagnosis of 21-OHD deficiency, including the immediate management and long-term implications. They were also given a clear explanation of how excess androgens produced by the enzyme deficiency affected the development of the baby's genitals. The parents' questions about future surgical options and the timing of surgery were answered.

In this case, the parents did not have any hesitation about raising their baby as female, and bonding with the baby seemed to be unhindered. The parents were taught the purpose of and how to administer the baby's medications. Mother and baby were discharged on day 3, with follow-up appointments scheduled with their pediatrician and pediatric endocrinologist. Although these parents initially expressed some anger and confusion related to the "change" in the baby's gender in the delivery room (from "it's a boy" to "we aren't sure"), they seemed to adjust fairly quickly to the change in gender, and even displayed a sense of humor about some aspects of the situation, such as their experience of expecting a boy for many weeks based on the prenatal sonogram and then finding out they had a girl. Although the parents did not make any firm decisions regarding genital surgery during the hospitalization, they planned to take the baby to a pediatric surgeon shortly after discharge for evaluation and consultation.

### *Discussion*

The extensively virilized neonate with CAH looks much, at first glance, like a male baby. It is not surprising that given that the parents, doctor, and nurses in this situation all expected a boy, no one immediately noticed the atypical genitals. Fortunately, this was detected quite early by the nurse performing the newborn examination. It is not unheard of for 46XX babies with significant virilization to be discharged from the hospital as boys only to be recalled by their pediatricians later when newborn screening results for CAH are positive. The signs and symptoms of adrenal decompensation in babies with salt-losing CAH usually manifest at 7 to 14 days of life; thus, most of these babies are identified by newborn screening tests before the onset of adrenal crisis.

## SUMMARY

Endocrine dysfunction may be somewhat less tangible and more mysterious than the more familiar problems we encounter in day-to-day care of neonates. We do not have monitors or rapid laboratory tests to evaluate the variations in functioning of the endocrine system. Given the potentially devastating consequences of endocrine disorders, however, health care professionals who work with newborns have a duty to broaden their basic knowledge and understanding of endocrine disease in this population. CAH is a well-described permanent endocrine disorder, and one that requires not only prompt recognition and management of the newborn but sensitivity, caring, and compassion when supporting the baby's family through this difficult period.

## REFERENCES

1. Kronenberg HM, Melmed S, Polonsky KS, et al, editors. Williams textbook of endocrinology. 11th edition. Philadelphia: Saunders Elsevier; 2008. p. 10.
2. Speiser PW. Molecular diagnosis of CYP21 mutations in congenital adrenal hyperplasia: implications for genetic counseling. Am J Pharmacogenomics 2001;1(2): 101–10.
3. Scott RR, Miller WL. Genetic and clinical features of P450 oxidoreductase deficiency. Horm Res 2008;69(5):266–75.

4. Riepe FG, Sippell WG. Recent advances in diagnosis, treatment, and outcome of congenital adrenal hyperplasia due to 21-hydroxylase deficiency. Rev Endocr Metab Disord 2007;8(4):349–63.
5. Miller WL, Achermann JC, Fluck CE. The adrenal cortex and its disorders. In: Sperling MA, editor. Pediatric endocrinology. 3rd edition. Philadelphia: Saunders Elsevier; 2008. p. 444–511.
6. Torresani T, Biason-Lauber A. Congenital adrenal hyperplasia: diagnostic advances. J Inherit Metab Dis 2007;30(4):563–75.
7. Witchel SF, Lee PA. Ambiguous genitalia. In: Sperling MA, editor. Pediatric endocrinology. 3rd edition. Philadelphia: Saunders Elsevier; 2008. p. 127–64.
8. Speiser PW. Congenital adrenal hyperplasia. In: Pescovitz OH, Eugster EA, editors. Pediatric endocrinology: mechanisms and management. Philadelphia: Lippincott, Williams & Wilkins; 2004. p. 600–20.
9. Kwon KT, Tsai VW. Metabolic emergencies. Emergency Med Clin N Am 2007; 25(4):1041–60.
10. Speiser PW, White PC. Congenital adrenal hyperplasia. N Engl J Med 2003; 349(8):776–88.
11. Parisi AM, Ramsdell LA, Burns MW, et al. A gender assessment team: experience with 250 patients over a period of 25 years. Genet Med 2007;9(6): 348–57.
12. National Newborn Genetics and Screening Resource Center. National Newborn Screening Status Report. 2008. Available at: http://genes-r-us.uthscsa.edu/nbsdisorders.htm. Accessed December 17, 2008.
13. Nordenstrom A, Ahmed S, Jones J, et al. Female preponderance in congenital adrenal hyperplasia due to CYP21 deficiency in England: implications for neonatal screening. Horm Res 2005;63(1):22–8.
14. Merke DP, Bornstein SR. Congenital adrenal hyperplasia. Lancet 2005; 365(9477):2125–36.
15. Reiner WG. Gender identity and sex-of-rearing in children with disorders of sexual differentiation. J Pediatr Endocrinol Metab 2005;18(6):549–53.
16. Houk CP, Lee PA. Consensus statement on terminology and management: disorders of sex development. Sex Dev 2008;2(4–5):172–80.
17. Mueller SC, Temple V, Oh E, et al. Early androgen exposure modulates spacial cognition in congenital adrenal hyperplasia. Psychoneuroendocrinology 2008; 33(7):973–80.
18. Manson JE. Prenatal exposure to sex steroid hormones and behavioral/cognitive outcomes. Metabolism 2008;57(Suppl 2):S16–21.
19. Crouch NS, Creighton SM. Minimal surgical intervention in the management of intersex conditions. J Pediatr Endocrinol Metab 2004;17(12):1591–6.
20. Luthra M, Hutson JM, Warne GL. Congenital adrenal hyperplasia in females with virilized genitalia: the problem of delayed diagnosis. J Paediatr Child Health 2008;24(4):254–7.
21. Speiser PW. Prenatal and neonatal diagnosis and treatment of congenital adrenal hyperplasia. Horm Res 2007;68(Suppl 5):90–2.
22. Sax L. How common is intersex? A response to Anne Fausto-Sterling. J Sex Res 2002;39(3):174–8.
23. Hughes IA. Disorders of sex development: a new definition and classification. Best Pract Res Clin Endocrinol Metab 2008;22(1):119–34.
24. Goto M, Hanley KP, Marcos J, et al. In humans, early cortisol biosynthesis provides a mechanism to safeguard female sexual development. J Clin Invest 2006;116(4):953–60.

25. White PC. Ontogeny of adrenal steroid biosynthesis: why girls will be girls. J Clin Invest 2006;116(4):872–4.
26. Consortium on the Management of Disorders of Sex Development. Clinical guidelines for the management of disorders of sex development in childhood. Intersex Society of North America, Rohnert Park, California. 2006. Available at: http://dsdguidelines.org/Accessed; Accessed December 17, 2008.
27. MacLellan DL, Diamond DA. Recent advances in external genitalia. Pediatr Clin North Am 2006;53:449–64.
28. Houk CP, Lee PA. Intersexed states: diagnosis and management. Endocrinol Metab Clin North Am 2005;34(3):791–810.
29. Hughes IA. Early management and gender assignment in disorders of sexual differentiation. Endocr Dev 2007;11:47–57.
30. Brown J, Warne G. Practical management of the intersex infant. J Pediatr Endocrinol Metab 2005;18:3–23.
31. Ogilvy-Stuart AL, Brain CE. Early assessment of ambiguous genitalia. Arch Dis Child 2004;89(5):401–7.

# Retinopathy of Prematurity

Debbie Fraser Askin, MN, RNC[a,b,c,*], William Diehl-Jones, RN, PhD[a,d]

**KEYWORDS**

- Retinopathy of prematurity • Eye disease
- Very low-birth-weight neonate • Premature • Newborn

Increasing survival rates for low birth weight infants have been accompanied in some cases by increasing rates of morbidities affecting survivors. One of these conditions, retinopathy of prematurity (ROP), targets the vascular system that supports the developing retina. Occurring almost exclusively in infants born at less than 32 weeks' gestation, the incidence of ROP in all premature infants is estimated to be 7.35%[1]

For many years, exposure to oxygen was believed to be the primary factor that lead to the development of abnormal blood vessel growth, scarring, and ultimately, retinal detachment. It is now apparent that oxygen exposure is not an absolute requirement for the development of ROP, and that this disease represents the response of an immature neonate to an environment that is markedly different from that of the uterus.

This article briefly reviews the history of ROP followed by a discussion of the pathogenesis of this complex disorder. We describe the International Classification System for ROP and identify risk factors and screening recommendations. Finally, we discuss some of the measures that have been used in an attempt to both prevent and treat ROP.

## HISTORY OF RETINOPATHY OF PREMATURITY

Originally known as "retrolental fibroplasia," ROP was first described by Terry[2] in 1942 and was responsible for an epidemic of blindness in the 1940s and 1950s. A study by Patz and colleagues[3] in 1952 and another by Kinsey[4] in 1956 showed the link between exposure to high concentrations of oxygen and the development of ROP, which led to restrictions in the use of oxygen. These restrictions decreased the incidence of

[a] Faculty of Nursing, University of Manitoba, Winnipeg, Manitoba, Canada
[b] Department of Pediatrics, Faculty of Medicine, University of Manitoba, Winnipeg, Manitoba, Canada
[c] St Boniface General Hospital, Winnipeg, Manitoba, Canada
[d] Department of Biological Sciences, Faculty of Science, University of Manitoba, Winnipeg, Manitoba, Canada
* Corresponding author. Faculty of Nursing, University of Manitoba, Winnipeg, MB R3T 2N2, Canada.
*E-mail address:* debbie_fraser@umanitoba.ca (D.F. Askin).

Crit Care Nurs Clin N Am 21 (2009) 213–233
doi:10.1016/j.ccell.2009.01.002 ccnursing.theclinics.com
0899-5885/09/$ – see front matter 

blindness in premature infants but resulted in a period of increased morbidity and mortality including cerebral palsy and lung disease.[5]

Technologic advances occurring in the late 1960s and early 1970s allowed for more precise measurements of blood oxygen levels; however, improving survival rates of low birth weight infants resulted in a resurgence of infants with ROP. In 1981, US estimates placed the number of infants at risk for blindness from ROP at 600 per year.[6] In 1991, data from a multicenter trial that studied 4099 infants weighing less than 1251 g reported on overall incidence of ROP of 65.8% and an incidence of 81.6% in infants weighing less than 1000 g.[7]

In the late 1990s, ROP remained the second leading cause of childhood blindness in developed countries.[8,9] More recent data from middle income countries, such as those in parts of South America, Eastern Europe, and Asia, suggest that the increase in cases of severe ROP has been even more substantial there, with an estimated 50,000 cases of blindness being reported.[10] So significant is the rate of ROP in middle income countries that some are referring to this as a third epidemic of ROP.[11] In these middle income countries, infants of higher birth weights are at greater risk of ROP development than those in higher income countries.[12,13]

Data from the Early Treatment for Retinopathy of Prematurity (ETROP) Cooperative Group published in 2005[14] compared current rates of ROP with those from the original Cryotherapy for ROP Cooperative Group (CRYO)[7] and found that rates of ROP were comparable—68% among infants of less than 1251 g in the ETROP study compared with 65.8%. The major change noted between the 2 studies is that, in the ETROP study, infants with more severe ROP were younger and smaller than those in the CRYO-ROP study (740 versus 831 g and 25.6 versus 26.5 weeks).[15] A similar review of infants born at less than 1250 g born between 1994 and 2000 found an increase in ROP over that time period (40%–54%) with a 2% to 5% rate of threshold ROP.[16]

Other published data suggest that recent changes in practice around oxygen administration and modifications in other treatment practices have resulted in a decrease in both the incidence and the severity of ROP.[17,18] These changes will be addressed below.

## CLASSIFICATION OF RETINOPATHY OF PREMATURITY

The International Classification System for Retinopathy of Prematurity (ICROP)[19] was first developed in 1984 by ophthalmologists from six countries, and was subsequently updated in 1987 and 2005. In 2006 practice guidelines, The American Academy of Pediatrics recommends the use of this classification system to describe and record retinal findings during screening examinations.[20] According to ICROP[19] the location of disease in the eye is first described according to the zone of the eye in which it occurs (**Fig. 1**). The amount of disease present is identified in terms of how many clock hours of the eye's circumference are affected. The zones reflect the central-to-peripheral pattern of blood vessel development and are identified as follows:

- *Zone I* extends from the optic nerve to twice the distance from the center of the optic nerve to the center of the macula.[19] ROP, which develops in zone I is of greatest concern because extensive scarring leading to retinal detachment is more likely in this location.
- *Zone II* extends from the edge of zone I to the nasal ora serrata found at the 3-o'clock position in the right eye and the 9-o'clock position in the left eye.[19]
- *Zone III* represents the last area of the retina to be vascularized and encompasses the remainder of the temporal retina.

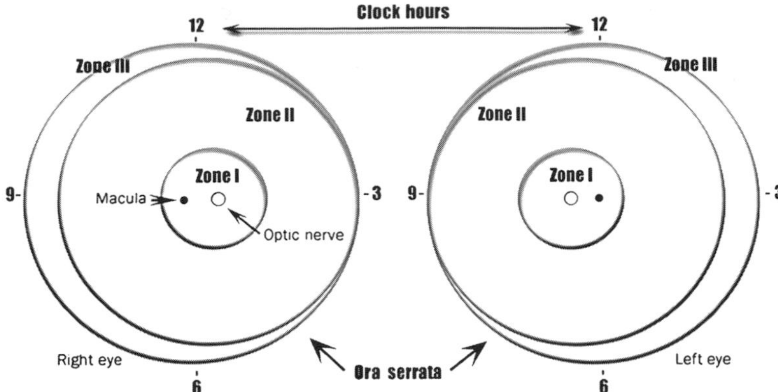


**Fig. 1.** Classification of ROP. (*From* American Academy of Pediatrics Section on Ophthalmology; American Academy of Ophthalmology; American Association for Pediatric Ophthalmology and Strabismus. Pediatrics 2006;117(2):573; with permission.)

Once the extent and area of the eye affected are identified, ROP is staged according to specific characteristic changes. Although it is not uncommon for more than one stage to be present in the eye, staging of the eye is based on the most severe stage present.[19]

- *Stage 1* ROP is characterized by a sharp white line of demarcation that lies flat against the retinal and marks the transitions between the vascular and avascular retina.
- *Stage 2* consists of a rolled ridge of scar tissue in the region of the white demarcation line. The length of the scar is variable. Small tuffs of new blood vessels called "popcorn" may be found behind the ridge.
- *Stage 3* is characterized by neovascularization originating from the posterior aspect of the ridge and growing into the vitreous. Stage 3 can further be subdivided into mild, moderate, or severe depending on the amount of new vessel growth projecting into the vitreous.
- *Stage 4* is subtotal retinal detachment caused by retraction or hardening of the scar tissue formed in earlier stages. Stage 4a is a partial detachment affecting the periphery of the retina. Stage 4b is a subtotal or total detachment involving the macula and fovea, usually with a fold extending through zones I, II, and III.
- *Stage 5* refers to a complete retinal detachment, with the retina assuming a closed or partially closed funnel from the optic nerve to the front of the eye.

### *Plus Disease*

Plus disease is present when, at any stage of ROP, the posterior veins are enlarged, and arterioles are tortuous (for example, stage 3+). Other findings of plus disease include poor papillary dilation and vitreous haze.[19] The presence of plus disease increases the likelihood that the disease will progress rapidly and significantly increases the chances of an unfavorable visual outcome.[21]

### *Pre-Plus Disease*

Pre-plus disease is a category added with the most recent revision of the ICROP classification system. The pre-plus designation is used when abnormal dilation and tortuosity of the vessels is present but not yet severe enough to be classed as plus disease. Pre-plus disease may progress to plus disease as dilation increases.[19]

In some infants greater than 1000 g, an unusually aggressive pattern of ROP, formerly termed "Rush disease," may occur. The newer term for this finding is "aggressive posterior ROP" or AP-ROP.[19] AP-ROP, most commonly seen in zone I, is characterized by ill-defined, dilated and tortuous vessels in the posterior portion of the eye. Shunts are present between the vessels, and hemorrhages may occur. AP-ROP does not progress through the usual stages, rather, untreated, it rapidly moves to severe ROP with retinal detachment.[22]

Threshold ROP is defined as extraretinal vascular proliferation found in zone 1 or 2 and encompassing a minimum of 5 uninterrupted clock hours or a total of 8 clock hours with plus disease. This risk of developing blindness in untreated threshold disease is 50%.[22] The designation of prethreshold ROP is used when the following findings are present: any ROP in zone 1; stage 2 ROP with plus disease or stage 3 without plus disease in zone 2; or stage 3 with plus disease but less than threshold.[23]

## PATHOGENESIS

### *Normal Retinal Development and Vascularization*

In utero, vascular development of the eye begins at approximately 6 weeks' gestation when the hyaloids artery fills the vitreous cavity with blood vessels. Vascularization of the retina begins at 14 to 16 weeks' gestation with the formation of spindle cells that begin developing at the optic nerve and form primitive vascular tubes. Spindle cells migrate from the area of the optic nerve to the nasal optic disc. Spindle cells do not migrate to the peripheral area of the retinal and normally disappear by 21 weeks' postmenstrual age.[13]

The second phase of normal retinal development is one of angiogenesis or the formation of new blood vessels from existing blood vessels. By 16 to 18 weeks of gestation, capillaries form at the edge of the peripheral retina and begin developing toward the periphery of the retina.[13] Vessel development is complete when it reaches the temporal ora serrata at approximately 40 to 44 weeks' gestation. Premature infants are born with incomplete vascularization of the retina. The area of the peripheral retina that is avascularized at birth is dependent on the infant's gestational age.[24]

Retinal development normally takes place in an intrauterine environment characterized by relative hypoxia with PaO2 levels of approximately 30 mm Hg and a saturation level of 70%.[25] This physiologic hypoxia is necessary to stimulate the production of growth factors that control blood vessel development.[26] To date, two factors have been identified that play a key role in normal vessel growth and, ultimately, in ROP. These are vascular endothelial growth factor (VEGF) and insulinlike growth factor (IGF-1). VEGF is a cytokine secreted by retinal astrocytes in response to hypoxia and found at the growing edge of the blood vessels in the retina.[13] Growth of the retina creates local hypoxia, which stimulates VEGF secretion, and blood vessels begin to grow toward the VEGF stimulus. As new blood vessels develop and oxygen is brought to the area of growth, VEGF secretion is suppressed until further growth again creates a condition of local hypoxia.[27]

The role of IGF-1 in retinal development is less clear, but it has been shown that the retinal vessels develop more slowly in the absence of IGF-1.[24] IGF-1 is initially supplied by the placenta and amniotic fluid, and levels decline after birth until endogenous production in the liver takes over.[24] Studies have found that IGF-1 levels are lowest in infants who later have ROP.[28,29]

### *Pathogenesis of Retinopathy of Prematurity*

ROP has been described as a two-phase process—the first phase characterized by cessation of normal blood vessel growth and the second phase by new blood vessel growth. These phases are described below:

#### *Phase1 retinopathy of prematurity*

The acute phase of ROP begins at 30 to 32 weeks' postmenstrual age and may develop slowly over time or, in the case of aggressive posterior ROP, may progress rapidly.[25] After birth, the premature infant's eye is exposed to an environment that, by intrauterine standards, is comparatively hyperoxic. Hyperoxia suppresses the secretion of VEGF leading to a cessation of normal vascular development, vasoconstriction of immature retinal vessels, and the death of some of the newly developed capillaries.[24,30] Although the mechanisms by which hyperoxia induce these changes are not fully known, it is speculated that the formation of reactive oxygen species (ROS), such as peroxynitrite, may be involved. Gu and colleagues[31] reported that hyperoxia-induced peroxynitrate triggers apoptosis in cultured retinal endothelial cells. Decreasing levels of IGF-1 also play a role in the cessation of vascular growth. Experimental models suggest that the presence of IGF-1 enhances the effects of VEGF on new blood vessel growth.[27] As the retina continues to grow, the nonvascularized area of the retina becomes hypoxic, leading to the second phase of ROP.

#### *Phase 2 retinopathy of prematurity*

Once a critical level of tissue hypoxia is reached, VEGF is secreted, leading to an angiogenic response and new vessel growth (neovascularization). Concurrently, increased production of IGF-1 may contribute to the development of new blood vessel growth by enhancing the effect VEGF on angiogenesis. As a result of increased VEGF secretion, a proliferation of new vessels form at the junction between the avascular and vascularized retina.

If circulation to the peripheral avascular retina can be re-established, ROP regresses, and excess vessels are reabsorbed. If the process is aggravated, neovascularization erupts into the vitreous, and vessel growth is uncontrolled. These vessels may regress and heal, but residual scarring causing a neovascular ridge may result. As scar tissue hardens and shrinks, it places traction on the retinal, which can lead to detachment.[25] Phase 2 ROP occurs between 32 and 34 weeks' postconception.[10]

Despite an increasing understanding of the pathogenesis of ROP, our current understanding of the disease does not fully explain the range of expression of the disease. The role of genetics, identification of the role of other growth factors, the contribution of oxidative stress and other cytokines such as those expressed in inflammation remain to be explored.

## RISK FACTORS

Despite extensive research examining the etiology of ROP, identifying which place neonates are at increased risk for ROP development has proven to be difficult. Studies in the late 1950s and 1960s suggested that prematurity or low birth weight and oxygen exposure were the most important contributors to the development of ROP.[10] These, along with illness severity, remain the major risk factors today.[24,32–34] Cases of ROP occurring during the 1970s and 1980s when oxygen administration was carefully controlled as well as reports of ROP occurring in premature infants not receiving supplemental oxygen suggest that, although oxygen is a risk factor, it is not the sole causative agent.[35–37]

### Oxygen

Studies from the 1950s first linked the use of oxygen therapy to the development of ROP.[3,38,39] It has been shown subsequently that normal retinal vascular development occurs through the expression of vasoendothelial growth factor in an environment of relative hypoxia,[26] making the link to exogenous oxygen plausible.

Despite the physiologic link between hyperoxia and suppression of VEGF, research has not been able to clearly delineate oxygen's role in the pathogenesis of ROP. Kinsey and colleagues[40] examined the relationship between arterial oxygen levels and ROP and failed to find a correlation with the incidence of ROP.[40] Similarly, a study using transcutaneous oxygen ($TcPO_2$) monitors to track blood oxygen levels found no difference in the incidence or severity of ROP for varying $TcPO_2$ levels in infants weighing less than 1000 g.[41] A case control study using rat pups done by Cunningham and colleagues[42] found that variability in transcutaneous oxygen levels in the first 2 weeks of life increased the risk for ROP while minimum or maximum total oxygen levels did not. Fluctuating PaO2 levels have also been found to increase the risk of threshold ROP in vulnerable infants.[43]

Support has been shown for the theory that duration of exposure to high oxygen levels is a factor in the development and severity of ROP.[42,44–47] One could speculate, however, that duration of oxygen therapy is also a marker for more significant illness, a factor that has also been linked to ROP development.[48]

Supplemental oxygen as a means to prevent progression of prethreshold ROP has been studied in large multicentered trial entitled "Supplemental Therapeutic Oxygen for Prethreshold Retinopathy of Prematurity" (STOP-ROP). STOP-ROP evaluated the safety and efficacy of maintaining oxygen saturations between 96% and 99% in low birth weight infants with ROP but found that this therapy did not reduce the severity of ROP and resulted in more adverse pulmonary complications. A small benefit was noted in infants with prethreshold ROP without plus disease when compared with those infants with plus disease, but this finding was not significant.[49] These findings were echoed in the systematic review conducted by Lloyd and colleagues[50] in 2003.

### Other Risk Factors

A wide range of other factors have been investigated in an attempt to explain the complex pathogenesis of ROP. These include blood transfusions, intraventricular hemorrhage, pneumothorax, mechanical ventilation, apnea, infection, hypercarbia, hypocarbia, patent ductus arteriosus, administration of prostaglandin synthetase inhibitors (indomethacin), vitamin E deficiency, light exposure, prenatal complications, and genetic factors.[25,36]

Intrauterine growth restriction and reduced postnatal growth have both been linked to ROP as has low serum levels of IGF-1.[51] Low levels of IGF-1 are found in infants with poor nutrition, poor weight gain, and other conditions, such as sepsis and necrotizing enterocolitis.[13]

Some early hypotheses regarding causation have not been supported by research findings. Both hypocarbia and hypercarbia have been disputed as correlates with ROP.[52–54] Animal models have suggested, however, that hypercarbia may increase blood flow to the retina, allowing greater delivery of oxygen to the tissues of the eye.[48,55,56] Fluctuating blood pressures were not found to contribute to the development of bronchopulmonary dysplasia[57] or prophylactic use of indomethacin for the treatment of a patent ductus arteriosus.[58,59] Research on the effect of surfactant therapy on the incidence of ROP has been mixed, with some studies finding a reduction in the severity of ROP,[60,61] and another study finding an overall increase in the rate of ROP in surfactant-treated neonates.[62]

Exposure to high levels of ambient light has been implicated in progression of ROP through the generation of oxygen free radicals, which damage the developing retinal blood vessels. Glass and coweorkers,[63] in 1985, reported a reduced incidence of ROP in neonates—especially those weighing less than 1000 g—exposed to reduced (150 lux) compared with standard (600 lux) lighting in the nursery. Other studies, including a large mulitcenter randomized, controlled trial, failed to find reduction in ROP as a result of reducing ambient light,[64–66] a finding confirmed by a later Cochrane review.[67]

Steroids may be administered either in the antenatal period or postnatal therapy for lung disease. Antenatal steroid administration has been found to reduce incidence of ROP,[68] whereas postnatal steroid exposure increases the risk of severe ROP.[69,70]

In many studies, factors found to correlate with a risk of ROP are also factors that reflect the severity of illness in the patient, and may or may not be directly linked to the development of ROP. Kim and colleagues[32] noted that apnea increases the risk of ROP development and also worsens pre-existing ROP. Akkoyun and associates[71] studied 88 infants less than 34 weeks of age and found that birth weight, blood transfusions, and duration of mechanical ventilation were correlated with the risk of ROP.

Blood transfusions were also cited as a risk factor in several other studies,[72–74] whereas Lui and others[75] identified birth weight of less than 1000 g, intraventricular hemorrhage, sepsis, and the use of dopamine or glucocorticoids as significant risk factors for ROP development in 159 infants weighing less than 1600 g at birth. Another review found that the primary risk factors for threshold ROP were maternal preeclampsia, birth weight, presence of pulmonary hemorrhage, and the duration of ventilation.[76]

Recent work highlights a possible genetic basis for both the development of ROP and in determining which infants progress to more severe disease. For example, ROP is more common in boys than in girls[77] and in Hispanic infants,[78] whereas white infants are more likely to have severe ROP than those of African American descent.[14] DNA studies have found genetic differences in the production of VGEF, which may explain why some infants progress to threshold disease while others do not.[79]

## SCREENING

Successful treatment of ROP is predicated on timely screening to identify those infants at risk of severe ROP. The American Academy of Pediatrics, the Academy of Ophthalmology, and the American Association for Pediatric Ophthalmology and Strabismus[20] have published screening guidelines that serve as the basis for national screening standards.

These joint screening guidelines make the following recommendations:[20]

- Screen all infants with a gestational age of less than 32 weeks or a birth weight of less than 1500 g
- Screen selected infants with a birth weight of 1500 to 2000 g who have had an unstable clinical course and are believed to be at high risk of ROP
- Examinations should be performed by a trained ophthalmologist
- Examinations should be initiated according to the infant's gestational and postnatal age (**Table 1**)

**Table 1**
**Timing of first eye examination based on gestational age at birth**

| | Age at Initial Examination, Wk | |
|---|---|---|
| **Gestational Age at Birth, Wk** | **Postmenstrual** | **Chronologic** |
| 22[a] | 31 | 9 |
| 23[a] | 31 | 8 |
| 24 | 31 | 7 |
| 25 | 31 | 6 |
| 26 | 31 | 5 |
| 27 | 31 | 4 |
| 28 | 32 | 4 |
| 29 | 33 | 4 |
| 30 | 34 | 4 |
| 31[b] | 35 | 4 |
| 32[b] | 36 | 4 |

Shown is a schedule for detecting prethreshold ROP with 99% confidence, usually well before any required treatment.

[a] This guideline should be considered tentative rather than evidence based for infants with a gestational age of 22 to 23 weeks, because of the small number of survivors in these gestational-age categories.

[b] If necessary.

*From* Section on Ophthalmology American Academy of Pediatrics; American Academy of Ophthalmology; American Association for Pediatric Ophthalmology and Strabismus. Pediatrics 2006;117(2):573; with permission.

- The timing of follow-up examinations is determined by the examining ophthalmologist and is based on the finding of the examination.

Follow-up examinations are usually done weekly when vascularization ends in zone 1 or the posterior area of zone 2, when there is any plus disease, or when there is stage 3 disease in any zone.[80] In the United Kingdom, ROP screening is discontinued when vascularization progresses to zone 3, at 37 weeks when no ROP has been detected, or when two successive examinations have shown regression of ROP. In the United States, screening is usually stopped when the infant reaches 45 weeks' postmenstrual age, when the entire retina is vascularized, or when the disease is regressing.[80]

Some issues regarding screening continue to be debated. With the recognition that aggressive AP-ROP in some extremely low birth weight infants (ELBW) occurs before 31 or 32 weeks of age[81] there is some concern that a delay in screening in this population will result in cases in which prethreshold disease is missed. This has prompted the revision of guidelines in the United Kingdom to recommend that infants born before 27 weeks' gestation have their first ROP screening when they reach 30 to 31 weeks' postmenstrual age.[82] Screening before 30 weeks' postmenstrual age is not recommended because the cornea is normally hazy at that age, making both examination and treatment difficult.[80]

A second area of debate centers on the question of whether screening could be limited to infants born at less than 30 weeks' gestation or 1251 g.[83,84] This is based on findings of studies such as the one done by Mathew and colleagues[83] who retrospectively reviewed the charts of 205 neonates born at less than 1500 g or 32 weeks' gestation to determine if screening criteria for ROP could be lowered to 1251 g or 30 weeks' gestational age. They found an overall incidence of ROP of 31.2% (64 infants), with 51 infants having stage 1 or 2 ROP. Ten infants had stage 3 ROP, and three had threshold disease; all of the more severe cases occurred in infants born at less than 28 weeks weighing less than 1000 g. Conversely, Hutchinson and colleagues[85] performed a retrospective review of 1118 infants with a birth weight of greater than 1250 g referred for ROP screening and identified 26 infants requiring laser therapy for ROP, including infants at 32 weeks' gestation and weighing up to 1874 g.

Given the importance of timely diagnosis and prompt intervention, it is critical that every neonatal intensive care unit have a program in place to identify infants who meet the ROP screening criteria. This includes a system to ensure that infants who are discharged home or transferred to another facility continue to receive timely and appropriate follow-up care. Ensuring that parents are aware of the importance of follow-up care is also an important part of any screening program.[20]

## PREVENTION

A wide variety of strategies have been investigated to prevent both development of ROP and the progression of the disease to more severe stages. Unfortunately, few of these strategies have been successful.

### *Preterm Birth*

Given that the single greatest risk factor in the development of ROP is prematurity, the prevention of preterm birth should be the overall goal. Work aimed at identifying strategies to prolong gestation while preventing fetal and maternal compromise will ultimately reduce the morbidity experienced in association with premature birth.

### *Controlling Oxygen Administration*

Until the role of oxygen in the pathogenesis of ROP is more clearly defined, hyperoxia and significant fluctuations in blood oxygen levels should be avoided. Several case control studies have been published that have shown a benefit when oxygen saturation levels have been regulated carefully.[17,86,87] In 2006, Vanderveen and colleagues[86] reported that lowering oxygen alarm limits to the range of 85% to 93% in infants weighing less than 1250 g resulted in a decrease in prethreshold ROP from 17.5% to 5.6%. No randomized, controlled trials have been published; however, a series of international randomized, controlled trial is now underway.[13]

Recommendations from these studies suggest that, for low birth weight infants, oxygen saturation be maintained between 85% and 93%.[17,86,87] Adjustments in the oxygen and ventilator settings should be made to keep oxygen saturations within acceptable levels while avoiding frequent changes in oxygen in response to brief variations in saturation levels.[17]

### *Nutrition*

Both intrapartum and postnatal growth failure have been found to increase the low birth weight infant's risk of ROP development. Prenatal strategies aimed at identifying growth-restricted infants, and, where possible, correcting deficits, should be addressed. Aggressive postnatal nutrition directed at preventing protein and calorie deficits is necessary because of the large number of low birth weight infants that do not achieve adequate weight gain in the first month of life.

### *Pharmacologic and Dietary Supplements*

A number of pharmacologic agents and dietary supplements have been examined to determine if they might play a role in the prevention of ROP. Several clinical and experimental studies have indicated that vitamin E (tocopherol) deficiency may cause ROP.[88–90] Several infant trials using vitamin E reported mixed results in terms of lowering the incidence and severity of ROP.[88,90,91] Increased rates of sepsis, necrotizing enterocolitis, intraventricular hemorrhage, and retinal hemorrhage in trials of high-dose intravenous vitamin E have prevented its adoption in practice.[90,92–94] More recently, a meta-analysis done by Brion and associates[95] found that vitamin E supplementation did reduce the risk of both ROP and intraventricular hemorrhage in very low birth weight infants but resulted in an increased risk of sepsis. These reviewers suggest that supplementation at high doses or resulting in levels greater than 3.5 mg/dL is not supported by evidence.

D-penicillamine is a potent antioxidant being studied for its role in preventing ROP. Lakatos and colleagues[96] identified a low incidence of ROP among the infants receiving D-penicillamine to prevent or treat hyperbilirubinemia. A meta-analysis of this and one other study[97] concluded that further investigation is warranted to determine if D-penicillamine reduces the incidence of acute ROP.[98] Subsequent to that recommendation, Christensen and colleagues[99] compared 15 premature infants treated with D-penicillamine with 34 matched controls and found that a 14-day course of D-penicillamine decreased the odds of ROP development from 60% to 21% with no short-term adverse effects noted. In infants with ROP, D-penicillamine did not reduce the need for surgery.

Inositol, a dietary supplement, has been studied as a means to reduce morbidity in premature infants with respiratory distress syndrome.[100,101] A significant reduction in stage 4 ROP was reported among infants receiving inositol in these studies. A Cochrane review of inositol suggests the need for randomized, controlled trials.[102]

Newer strategies for pharmacologic treatment await further testing and development. In an animal model of ROP, Saito and colleagues[103] report that apocyanin, and inhibitor of nicotinamide adenine dinucleotide phosphate (NAPDH) oxidase (which is involved in peroxynitrate formation), inhibits apoptosis of retinal cells and avascularization. This poses the possibility of using apocyanin or other NADPH oxidase inhibitors in adjuvant therapies to treat ROP. In a more recent study, Geissen and others[104] report that, in a similar animal model of ROP, intravitreous injection of a neutralizing antibody to VEGF reduces intravitreous neovascularization, while not interfering with intraretinal vascularization. Again, this offers a treatment for severe ROP, when other courses fail.

## TREATMENT

Cryotherapy using a liquid nitrogen probe and laser treatment using argon or infrared diode laser have been used to successfully treat ROP. The exact mechanism by which these treatments work is unclear, but it is believed that destroying avascular tissue on the retina reduces the release of angiogenic factors leading to a reduction in vascular proliferation.[105,106]

In the past, cryotherapy or laser ablation was done when the criteria for threshold disease was met. More recently, intervention in the prethreshold stage of ROP has been shown to result in better visual outcomes than treatment at threshold disease.[107] In the ETROP study, unfavorable visual acuity outcomes were reduced from 19.5% to 14.5%, and unfavorable structural outcomes were reduced to 9.1%. Infants in the early treatment group did experience more apnea and bradycardia and had a higher rate of reintubation, perhaps reflecting the younger age at which treatment took place. In a retrospective review done by Alme and associates,[18] it was noted that the incidence of retinal detachment before the change in treatment guidelines was 10.3%

compared with 1.9% after the change in guidelines, despite the second group having a lower birth weight and gestational age.

The American Academy of Pediatrics Section on Ophthalmology; the American Academy of Ophthalmology; and the American Association for Pediatric Ophthalmology and Strabismus Guidelines[20] now recommend intervention when ROP meets the following criteria: zone I ROP at any stage when plus disease is present, stage 3 ROP in zone I in the absence of plus disease, or stage 2 or 3 ROP in zone II with plus disease.

There is still some debate in the literature surrounding the adoption of these treatment criteria. The diagnosis of plus disease is subjective, and significant differences in its diagnosis have been identified in research examining congruence among expert ophthalmologists.[108] Work is ongoing to develop computerized programs to more accurately diagnosis the presence of pre-plus and plus disease.[109–111] There is also discussion in the literature that suggests that these recommendations may result in the treatment of some infants whose disease would have regressed spontaneously.[112]

### *Cryotherapy*

Cryotherapy, used to freeze the avascular area of the retina anterior to the area of disease, was introduced in the 1960s.[113] Cryotherapy remained the primary form of ROP treatment for a number of years but has now been largely replaced by laser ablation. Cryotherapy is currently used in cases in which blood or corneal haziness obscures the view of the retina making it impossible to use laser treatment.[114]

The benefits of cryotherapy for treatment of threshold ROP was shown by a large multicenter trial that enrolled 9751 infants with birth weights of less than 1251 g in 23 US centers. Enrollment in the CRYO-ROP study was ended early because a significant benefit to treatment with cryotherapy was found.[115] In this study, threshold ROP developed in 291 infants (6%), who were randomly assigned to either the control group or treated with cryotherapy within 72 hours of diagnosis. Cryotherapy was shown to significantly reduce the incidence of unfavorable visual outcomes, such as posterior retinal detachment, a retinal fold involving the macula or rotrolental tissue. Poor visual outcomes occurred in 31.1% of treated eyes compared with 51.4% of control eyes at 3 months[116] and in 25.7% of treated eyes compared with 47.4% of control eyes at 1 year. Functional outcomes measured 1 year after treatment suggested that 35% of treated eyes had an unfavorable functional outcome compared with 56.3% in untreated eyes.[117]

These results persisted at the 10-year follow-up for unfavorable distance visual acuity: 44.4% in treated eyes versus 62.1% control eyes and for fundus status (27.2% versus 47.9%). Over the 10-year follow-up period, the number of retinal detachments in the control eyes increased to 41.4%, whereas detachments in the treated eyes remained at 22%.[118]

### *Laser Photocoagulation*

In the last 15 years, laser ablation therapy has almost completely replaced cryotherapy in the treatment of most cases of ROP. Compared with cryotherapy, laser treatment is less traumatic to surrounding tissues, causes less discomfort, and is more effective in areas of the eye that are difficult to access such as zone 1. Laser treatment also has a lower incidence of associated complications, including intraocular hemorrhage.[119]

Research comparing laser therapy with cryotherapy has shown that eyes treated with laser photocoagulation have better structural and functional outcomes. In a 10-year follow-up study of 44 eyes (25 patients) Ng and colleagues[120] found that retinal dragging was 7.2 times more likely to occur in cryotherapy-treated eyes compared with eyes treated with laser therapy and that retinal dragging increased the risk of poor visual outcomes. Myopia was also significantly more likely to occur in cryotherapy-treated eyes than in eyes treated with laser therapy.[121] In a similar study, Paysse and associates[122] compared results of a retrospective chart review of 63 infants receiving cryotherapy with 70 infants receiving laser treatment. Results showed that resolution of ROP was achieved in 56.4% of the cryotherapy group compared with 87.5% of the laser group. Visual acuity in the cryotherapy group averaged 20/103 compared with 20/49 in the laser group. These findings have been verified by a number of studies showing the efficacy of laser ablation in the treatment of ROP,[123–127] including a Cochrane systematic review.[128]

Complications of laser treatment include burns to the cornea iris or lens, retinal hemorrhage, and rupture of the choroid.[22] Use of laser therapy has been found to increase the risk of cataract development;[129] however, when diode red laser is used, the risk of cataracts is lower than with argon green lasers.[130]

### *Treatment for Retinal Detachment*

Two treatments, both with limited success, have been used to manage retinal detachment after ROP. Scleral buckling (SB), which involves the placement of a silicone band around the eye, alters the shape of the eye, and pushes the retinal back toward the rear wall of the eye where it can reattach. Resulting visual acuity has been reported to range from 20/60 to 18/400[131] with severe myopia, anisometropia, and amblyopia reported as complications.[22] The poor success rate of SB is attributed to the fact that this procedure does not alter the traction forces applied by the scar tissue within the eye. Additionally, a second procedure is required at a later date to remove the band so that the eye can continue to grow.[22]

Vitrectomy with or without scleral buckling is also used to treat retinal detachment. A lens-sparing vitrectomy (LVS) involves removal of the vitreous and scar tissue, allowing the retinal to contact the posterior wall of the eye. The rate of anatomic reattachment of the macula is reported to be approximately 90% compared with rates of 60% to 75% for SB.[132–136] Functional results are more variable, with one study reporting on 45 eyes with stage 4A retinopathy treated with vitrectomy in which visual acuity was 20/80 or better in 38 of the treated eyes.[137]

In follow-up of infants in the ETROP study who underwent vitrectomy or scleral buckling, macular attachment was achieved in 16 of 48 eyes. Nine months after treatment, 30% of eyes treated with vitrectomy with or without scleral buckling had macular attachment, whereas macular attachment occurred in 60% of eyes treated with scleral buckling alone. In 11 eyes, all with stage 5 ROP, some successes occurred in terms of macular reattachment, but all had poor visual outcome, with six eyes having no light perception, three having light perception only, and two with reduced vision.[138] It is speculated that infants in the ETROP study had a more aggressive form of ROP, which may account for the difference in success rates compared with those seen in other studies.[106] Some clinicians use a combination of the two procedures (LVS and SB); however, findings from a recent study suggest that the addition of SB does not increase the rate of macular reattachment.[139]

Reported complications of LSV include retinal tears, cataracts, and glaucoma. The incidence of cataracts is reported to be 5% to 15% after vitrectomy.[140,141] Poor outcomes for all surgical interventions are predicted by the presence of plus disease, vitreous haze, and continued neovascularization.[142]

### *Investigational Therapies*

The recognition of the role of VGEF in the development of abherant vascular issues in ROP has led to research using VEGF inhibitors to prevent new blood vessel growth in

ROP-affected eyes. One of these blockers, bevacizumab, a monoclonal antibody, had been used to treat diabetic retinopathy[143,144] and macular degeneration in adults.[145] Case reports of these drugs used in rescue treatment for severe ROP have been published with promising results.[145–147]

## PROGNOSIS

Visual outcome in ROP is dependent on the stage and location of the disease. The greatest impact on vision is seen when ROP involves the macula. Stage 1 and 2 disease are usually confined to the peripheral retina and resolve spontaneously without scarring.[148] These infants do, however, remain at higher risk for the development of myopia, amblyopia, astigmatism, strabismus and glaucoma,[30] and vitreous hemorrhage.[149] Late retinal degeneration and retinal detachments have also been reported in teens and adults with mild forms of ROP.[150,151]

Untreated ROP that reaches stage 3 or 4 poses a significant risk for visual impairment, because tension is placed on the retinal as the scar tissue shrinks and retracts. Infants treated for stage 3 or 4 disease have unfavorable structural outcomes in approximately 3% of cases and unfavorable functional outcome in 5% of cases. These poor outcomes are more likely to be associated with zone 1 ROP or ROP in more than 6 clock hours in zone 2.[152] In cases of stage 4b or 5 ROP, retinal funneling or detachment results in blindness. Blindness occurs in about 50% of eyes with untreated threshold disease.[98]

## SUMMARY

A significant amount of research has been done in an attempt to shed light on both the pathogenesis of ROP and on strategies for its prevention and treatment. Recent changes in the criteria for treatment as well as tighter control of oxygen saturation and improvements in postnatal nutrition have reduced the incidence and severity of ROP. Much work remains to further elucidate the role of vasogenic factors, such as VEGF and IGF and to determine the role of exogenous antagonists and gene therapies aimed at controlling the process of vascularization of the retinal. Until this work is complete, nurses will continue to play an integral role in modulating the environment of the very low birth weight infant.

## REFERENCES


1. Lad EM, Nguyen TC, Morton JM, et al. Retinopathy of prematurity in the United States. Br J Ophthalmol 2008;92(3):320–5.
2. Terry TL. Extreme prematurity and fibroblastic overgrowth of persistent vascular sheath behind each crystalline lens. Am J Ophthalmol 1942;25(2):203–4.
3. Patz A, Hoeck LE, DeLaCruz E. Studies on the effect of high oxygen administration in retrolental fibroplasia. I. Nursery observations. Am J Ophthalmol 1952;35:1248–53.
4. Kinsey VE. Cooperative study of retrolental fibroplasia and the use of oxygen. Arch Ophthalmol 1956;56:481–543.
5. Cross KW. Cost of preventing retrolental fibroplasia? Lancet 1973;2(835):954–6.
6. Phelps DL. Retinopathy of prematurity: an estimate of visual loss in the United States. Pediatrics 1981;67(6):924–5.
7. Palmer EA, Flynn JT, Hardy RJ, et al. Incidence and early course of retinopathy of prematurity. The Cryotherapy for Retinopathy of Prematurity Cooperative Group. Ophthalmology 1991;98(11):1628–40.

8. Steinkuller PG, Du L, Gilbert C, et al. Childhood blindness. J AAPOS 1999;3(1): 26–32.
9. Gilbert C, Rahi J, Eckstein M, et al. Retinopathy of prematurity in middle-income countries. Lancet 1997;350(9070):12–4.
10. Saugstad OD. Oxygen and retinopathy of prematurity. J Perinatol 2006;26:S46–50.
11. Gilbert C. Retinopathy of prematurity: a global perspective of the epidemics, population of babies at risk and implications for control. Early Hum Dev 2008; 84(2):77–82.
12. Gilbert C, Fielder A, Gordillo L, et al. International NO-ROP Group. Characteristics of infants with severe retinopathy of prematurity in countries with low, moderate, and high levels of development: implications for screening programs. Pediatrics 2005;115(5):e518–25.
13. Fleck BW, McIntosh N. Pathogenesis of retinopathy of prematurity and possible preventative strategies. Early Hum Dev 2008;84:83–8.
14. Good WV, Hardy RJ, Dobson V, et al. Early Treatment for Retinopathy of Prematurity Cooperative Group. The incidence and course of retinopathy of prematurity: findings from the early treatment for retinopathy of prematurity study. Pediatrics 2005;116(1):15–23.
15. Hardy RJ, Palmer EA, Dobson V, et al. Risk analysis of prethreshold ROP. Arch Ophthalmol 2003;121:1699–701.
16. O'Connor MT, Vohr BR, Tucker R, et al. Is retinopathy of prematurity increasing among infants less than 1250 g birthweight? J Perinatol 2003;23(8):673–8.
17. Chow LC, Wright KW, Sola A, CSMC Oxygen Administration Study Group. Can changes in clinical practice decrease the incidence of severe retinopathy of prematurity in very low birth weight infants? Pediatrics 2003;111(2):339–45.
18. Alme AM, Mulhern ML, Hejkal TW, et al. Outcome of retinopathy of prematurity patients following adoption of revised indications for treatment. BMC Ophthalmol 2008;8(1):23.
19. International Committee for the Classification of Retinopathy of Prematurity. The International classification of retinopathy of prematurity revisited. Arch Ophthalmol 2005;123(7):991–9.
20. American Academy of Pediatrics Section on Ophthalmology, American Academy of Ophthalmology, American Association for Pediatric Ophthalmology and Strabismus. Screening examination of premature infants for retinopathy of prematurity. Pediatrics 2006;117(2):572–6.
21. Schaffer DB, Palmer EA, Plotsky DF, et al. Prognostic factors in the natural course of retinopathy of prematurity. The Cryotherapy for Retinopathy of Prematurity Cooperative Group. Ophthalmology 1993;100(2):230–7.
22. Clark D, Mandal K. Treatment of retinopathy of prematurity. Early Hum Dev 2008; 84:95–9.
23. William VG, Early Treatment for Retinopathy of Prematurity Cooperative Group. Final results of the Early Treatment for Retinopathy of Prematurity (ETROP) randomized trial. Trans Am Ophthalmol Soc 2004;102:233–48.
24. Smith LE. Pathogenesis of retinopathy of prematurity. Semin Neonatol 2003;8: 469–73.
25. Chen J, Smith LE. Retinopathy of prematurity. Angiogenesis 2007;10(2):133–40.
26. Chan-Ling T, Gock B, Stone J. Supplemental oxygen therapy: basis for noninvasive treatment of retinopathy of prematurity. Invest Ophthalmol Vis Sci 1995;36: 1215–30.
27. Smith LE. Pathogenesis of retinopathy of prematurity. Acta Paediatr Suppl 2002; 91(437):26–8.

28. Smith LE, Shen W, Perruzzi C, et al. Regulation of vascular endothelial growth factor-dependent retinal neovascularization by insulin-like growth factor-1 receptor. Nat Med 1999;5:1390–95.
29. Hellstrom A, Pernuzzi C, Ju M, et al. Low IGF-1 suppresses VEGF-a survival signaling in retinal endothelial cells: direct correlation with clinical retinopathy of prematurity. Proc Natl Acad Sci U S A 2001;98:5804–8.
30. Stout AU, Stout JT. Retinopathy of prematurity. Pediatr Clin North Am 2003;50(1): 77–87.
31. Gu XG, El-Remessy AB, Brooks SE, et al. Hyperoxia induces retinal vascular endothelial cell apoptosis through formation of peroxynitrite. Am J Physiol, Cell Physiol 2003;285:C546–54.
32. Kim TI, Sohn J, Pi SY, et al. Postnatal risk factors of retinopathy of prematurity. Paediatr Perinat Epidemiol 2004;18(2):130–4.
33. Quinn GE. The 'ideal' management of retinopathy of prematurity. Eye 2005; 19(10):1044–9.
34. Tasman W, Patz A, McNamara JA, et al. Retinopathy of prematurity: the life of a lifetime disease. Am J Ophthalmol 2006;141(1):167–74.
35. Flynn JT. Acute proliferative retrolental fibroplasia: multivariate risk analysis. Trans Am Ophthalmol Soc 1983;81:549–91.
36. Lucey JF, Dangman B. A reexamination of the role of oxygen in retrolental fibroplasia. Pediatrics 1984;73(1):82–96.
37. Buksh MJ, Dai S, Kuschel CA. AP-ROP in an infant with minimal oxygen exposure. Paediatr Child Health 2008;44(4):228–30.
38. Campbell K. Intensive oxygen therapy as a possible cause of retrolental fibroplasias: a clinical approach. Med J Aust 1951;2:48–50.
39. Ashton N, Cook C. Direct observation of the effect of oxygen on developing vessels: preliminary report. Br J Ophthalmol 1954;38:433–40.
40. Kinsey VE, Arnold HJ, Kalina RE, et al. $PaO_2$ levels and retrolental fibroplasia: a report of the cooperative study. Pediatrics 1977;60(5):655–68.
41. Bancalari E, Flynn J, Goldberg RN, et al. Influence of transcutaneous oxygen monitoring on the incidence of retinopathy of prematurity. Pediatrics 1987; 79(5):663–9.
42. Cunningham S, Fleck BW, Elton RA, et al. Transcutaneous oxygen levels in retinopathy of prematurity. Lancet 1995;346:1464–5.
43. York JR, Landers S, Kirby RS, et al. Arterial oxygen fluctuation and retinopathy of prematurity in very-low-birth-weight infants. J Perinatol 2004;24(2):82–7.
44. Flynn JT, Bancalari E, Snyder ES, et al. A cohort study of transcutaneous oxygen tension and the incidence and severity of retinopathy of prematurity. N Engl J Med 1992;326(16):1050–4.
45. Hesse L, Eberl W, Schlaud M. Blood transfusion. Iron load and retinopathy of prematurity. Eur J Pediatr 1997;156:465–70.
46. Batton DG, Roberts C, Trese M. Severe retinopathy of prematurity and steroid exposure. Pediatrics 1992;90:534–6.
47. Gallo JE, Jacobsen L, Broberger U. Perinatal factors associated with retinopathy of prematurity. Acta Paediatr Scand 1993;82:829–34.
48. McColm JR, Fleck BW. Retinopathy of prematurity: causation. Semin Neonatol 2001;6:453–60.
49. STOP-ROP Multicenter Study Group. Supplemental Therapeutic Oxygen for Prethreshold Retinopathy Of Prematurity (STOP-ROP), a randomized, controlled trial. I: primary outcomes. Pediatrics 2000;105(2):295–310.

50. Lloyd J, Askie L, Smith J, et al. Supplemental oxygen for the treatment of prethreshold retinopathy of prematurity. Cochrane Database Syst Rev 2003;(2): CD003482.
51. Hellström A, Engström E, Hård AL, et al. Postnatal serum insulin-like growth factor I deficiency is associated with retinopathy of prematurity and other complications of premature birth. Pediatrics 2003;112(5):1016–20.
52. Brown DR, Milley JR, Ripepi UJ. Retinopathy of prematurity. Risk factors in a five-year cohort of critically ill premature neonates. Am J Dis Child 1987;141:154–60.
53. Mariani G, Cifuentes J, Carlo WA. Randomised trial of permissive hypercapnia in preterm infants. Pediatrics 1999;104:1082–8.
54. Gellen B, McIntosh N, McColm JR. Is the partial pressure of carbon dioxide in the blood related to the development of retinopathy of prematurity? Br J Ophthalmol 2001;85:1044–5.
55. Berkowitz BA. Adult and newborn rat inner retinal oxygenation during carbogen and 100% oxygen breathing. Invest Ophthalmol Vis Sci 1996;37:2089–98.
56. Stiris T, Odden JP, Hansen TW, et al. The effect of arterial PCO2-variations on ocular and cerebral blood flow in the newborn piglet. Pediatr Res 1989;25: 205–8.
57. Cunningham S, Symon AG, Elton RA. Intra-arterial blood pressure reference ranges, death and morbidity in very low birthweight infants during the first seven days of life. Early Hum Dev 1999;56:151–65.
58. Schmidt B, Davis P, Moddemann D. Long-term effects of indomethacin prophylaxis in extremely low-birth-weight infants. N Engl J Med 2001;344: 1966–72.
59. Knight DB. The treatment of patent ductus arteriosus in preterm infants. A review and overview of randomized trials. Semin Neonatol 2001;6:63–73.
60. Termote J, Schalij-Delfos NE, Brouwers HA, et al. New developments in neonatology: less severe retinopathy of prematurity? J Pediatr Ophthalmol Strabismus 2000;37:142–8.
61. Penn JS, Rajaratnam VS, Collier RJ. The effect of an angiostatic steroid on neovascularization in a rat model of retinopathy of prematurity. Invest Ophthalmol Vis Sci 2001;42:283–90.
62. Termote JU, Schalij-Delfos NE, Wittebol-Post D, et al. Surfactant replacement therapy: a new risk factor in developing retinopathy of prematurity? Eur J Pediatr 1994;153:113–6.
63. Glass P, Avery GB, Subramanian KN, et al. Effect of bright light in the hospital nursery on the incidence of retinopathy of prematurity. N Engl J Med 1985; 313(7):401–4.
64. Hommura S, Usuki Y, Takei K, et al. Ophthalmologic care of very low birth weight infants. Report 4. clinical studies of the influence of light on the incidence of retinopathy of prematurity. Nippon Ganka Gakkai Zasshi 1988;92(3):456–61.
65. Ackerman B, Sherwonit E, Williams J. Reduced incidental light exposure effect on the development of retinopathy of prematurity in low birth weight infants. Pediatrics 1989;83(6):958–62.
66. Reynolds JD, Hardy RJ, Kennedy KA, et al. Lack of efficacy of light reduction in preventing retinopathy of prematurity. Light Reduction in Retinopathy of Prematurity (LIGHT-ROP) Cooperative Group. N Engl J Med 1998;338(22):1572–6.
67. Phelps DL, Watts JL. Early light reduction for preventing retinopathy of prematurity in very low birth weight infants. Cochrane Database Syst Rev 2001;(1): CD000122.

68. Console V, Gagliardi L, De Giorgi A. Retinopathy of prematurity and antenatal corticosteroids. The Italian ROP Study Group. Acta Biomed Ateneo Parmense 1997;68:75–9.
69. Haroon PM, Dhanireddy R. Association of postnatal dexamethasone use and fungal sepsis in the development of severe retinopathy of prematurity and progression to laser therapy in extremely low-birth-weight infants. J Perinatol 2001;21:242–7.
70. Halliday HL, Ehrenkranz RA. Delayed (>3 weeks) postnatal corticosteroids for chronic lung disease in preterm infants. [Cochrane Review]. Cochrane Database Syst Rev 2001;(2):CD001145.
71. Akkoyun I, Oto S, Yilmaz G, et al. Risk factors in the development of mild and severe retinopathy of prematurity. J AAPOS 2006;10(5):449–53.
72. Dutta S, Narang S, Narang A, et al. Risk factors of threshold retinopathy of prematurity. Indian Pediatr 2004;41(7):665–71.
73. Cooke RW, Clark D, Hickey-Dwyer M, et al. The apparent role of blood transfusions in the development of retinopathy of prematurity. Eur J Pediatr 1993;152: 833–6.
74. Dani C, Reali MF, Bertini G. The role of blood transfusions and iron intake on retinopathy of prematurity. Early Hum Dev 2001;62:57–63.
75. Liu PM, Fang PC, Huang CB, et al. Risk factors of retinopathy of prematurity in premature infants weighing less than 1600 g. Am J Perinatol 2005;22(2): 115–20.
76. Shah VA, Yeo CL, Ling YL, et al. Incidence, risk factors of retinopathy of prematurity among very low birth weight infants in Singapore. Ann Acad Med Singap 2005;34(2):169–78.
77. Csak K, Szabo V, Szabo A, et al. Pathogenesis and genetic basis for retinopathy of prematurity. Front Biosci 2006;1(11):908–20.
78. Chiang MF, Arons RR, Flynn JT, et al. Incidence of retinopathy of prematurity from 1996 to 2000: analysis of a comprehensive New York state patient database. Ophthalmology 2004;111(7):1317–25.
79. Cooke RW, Drury JA, Mountford R, et al. Genetic polymorphisms and retinopathy of prematurity. Invest Ophthalmol Vis Sci 2004;45(6):1712–5.
80. O'Keefe M, Kirwan C. Screening for retinopathy of prematurity. Early Hum Dev 2008;84:89–94.
81. Subhani M, Combs A, Weber P, et al. Screening guidelines for retinopathy of prematurity: the need for revision in extremely low birth weight infants. Pediatrics 2001;107(4):656–9.
82. Royal College of Paediatrics & Child Health & Royal College of Ophthalmologists. UK retinopathy of Prematurity Guideline. 2007. Available at: http://www.rcophth.ac.uk/docs/publications/ROP_Guideline_-_Masterv11-ARF-2.pdf. Accessed November 28, 2008.
83. Mathew MR, Fern AI, Hill R. Retinopathy of prematurity: are we screening too many babies? Eye 2002;16(5):538–42.
84. Ho SF, Mathew MR, Wykes W, et al. Retinopathy of prematurity: an optimum screening strategy. J AAPOS 2005;9(6):584–8.
85. Hutchinson AK, O'Neil JW, Morgan EN, et al. Retinopathy of prematurity in infants with birth weights greater than 1250 grams. J AAPOS 2003;7(3):190–4.
86. VanderVeen DK, Mansfield TA, Eichenwald EC. Lower oxygen saturation alarm limits decrease the severity of retinopathy of prematurity. J AAPOS 2006;10(5): 445–8.

87. Coe K, Butler M, Reavis N, et al. Special Premie Oxygen Targeting (SPOT): a program to decrease the incidence of blindness in infants with retinopathy of prematurity. J Nurs Care Qual 2006;21(3):230–5.
88. Milner RA, et al. Vitamin E supplement in under 1,500 gram neonates. Retinopathy of Prematurity Conference. Columbus (OH): Ross Laboratories; 1981. p. 703–16.
89. Finer NN, Schindler RF, Grant G, et al. Effect of intramuscular vitamin E on frequency and severity of retrolental fibroplasia: a controlled trial. Lancet 1982;1(8281):1087–91.
90. Johnson L, Quinn GE, Abbasi S, et al. Effect of sustained pharmacologic vitamin E levels on incidence and severity of retinopathy of prematurity: a controlled clinical trial. J Pediatr 1989;114(5):827–38.
91. Raju TN, Langenberg P, Bhutani V, et al. Vitamin E prophylaxis to reduce retinopathy of prematurity: a reappraisal of published trials. J Pediatr 1997;131(6): 844–50.
92. Rosenbaum AL, Phelps DL, Isenberg SJ, et al. Retinal hemorrhage in retinopathy of prematurity associated with tocopherol treatment. Ophthalmology 1985;92(8):1012–4.
93. Phelps DL, Rosenbaum AL, Isenberg SJ, et al. Tocopherol efficacy and safety for preventing retinopathy of prematurity: a randomized, controlled, double-masked trial. Pediatrics 1987;79(4):489–500.
94. Ehrenkranz RA. Vitamin E and retinopathy of prematurity: still controversial. J Pediatr 1989;114(5):801–3.
95. Brion LP, Bell EF, Raghuveer TS. Vitamin E supplementation for prevention of morbidity and mortality in preterm infants. Cochrane Database Syst Rev 2003;(4):CD003665.
96. Lakatos L, Hatvani I, Oroszlan G, et al. Controlled trial of D-penicillamine to prevent retinopathy of prematurity. Acta Paediatr Hung 1986;27:47–56.
97. Lakatos L, Lakatos Z, Hatvani I, et al. Controlled trial of use of D-Penicillamine to prevent retinopathy of prematurity in very low-birth-weight infants. In: Stern L, Oh W, Friis-Hansen B, editors. Physiologic foundations of perinatal care. St. Louis: Elsevier; 1987. p. 9–23.
98. Phelps DL, Lakatos L, Watts JL. D-Penicillamine for preventing retinopathy of prematurity in preterm infants. Cochrane Database Syst Rev 2001;(1): CD001073.
99. Christensen RD, Alder SC, Richards SC, et al. D-Penicillamine administration and the incidence of retinopathy of prematurity. J Perinatol 2007;27(2): 103–11.
100. Hallman M, Jarvanpaa AL, Pohjavuori M. Respiratory distress syndrome and inositol supplementation in preterm infants. Arch Dis Child 1986;61:1076–83.
101. Hallman M, Bry K, Hoppu K, et al. Inositol supplementation in premature infants with respiratory distress syndrome. N Engl J Med 1992;326(19):1233–9.
102. Howlett A, Ohlsson A. Inositol for respiratory distress syndrome in preterm infants. Cochrane Database Syst Rev 2003;(4):CD000366.
103. Saito Y, Geisen P, Uppal A, et al. Inhibition of NAD(P)H oxidase reduces apoptosis and avascular retina in an animal model of retinopathy of prematurity. Mol Vis 2008;13:840–53.
104. Geisen P, Peterson LJ, Martiniuk D, et al. Neutralizing antibody to VEGF reduces intravitreous neovascularization and may not interfere with ongoing intraretinal vascularization in a rat model of retinopathy of prematurity. Mol Vis 2008;14: 345–57.

105. Steinmetz RL, Brooks HL Jr. Diode laser photocoagulation to the ridge and avascular retina in threshold retinopathy of prematurity. Retina 2002;22(1): 48–52.
106. Hubbard GB 3rd. Surgical management of retinopathy of prematurity. Curr Opin Ophthalmol 2008;19(5):384–90.
107. Early Treatment For Retinopathy Of Prematurity Cooperative Group. Revised indications for the treatment of retinopathy of prematurity: results of the early treatment for retinopathy of prematurity randomized trial. Arch Ophthalmol 2003;121(12):1684–94.
108. Wallace DK, Quinn GE, Freedman SF, et al. Agreement among pediatric ophthalmologists in diagnosing plus and preplus disease in retinopathy of prematurity. J AAPOS 2008;12(4):352–6.
109. Johnson KS, Mills MD, Karp KA, et al. Semiautomated analysis of retinal vessel diameter in retinopathy of prematurity patients with and without plus disease. Am J Ophthalmol 2007;143:723–5.
110. Wallace DK, Freedman SF, Zhao Z, et al. Accuracy of ROPtool vs individual examiners in assessing retinal vascular tortuosity. Arch Ophthalmol 2007;125: 1523–30.
111. Swanson C, Cocker KD, Parker KH, et al. Semiautomated computer analysis of vessel growth in preterm infants without and with ROP. Br J Ophthalmol 2003;87: 1474–7.
112. Coats D, Saunders R. The dilemma of exercising clinical judgment in the treatment of retinopathy of prematurity. Arch Ophthalmol 2005;123:408–9.
113. Fielder AR. Cryotherapy of retinopathy of prematurity. In: Davidson SI, Jay B, editors. Recent advances in ophthalmology, vol 8. Edinburgh (UK): Churchill Livingstone; 1992. p. 129–48.
114. Hutcheson KA. Retinopathy of prematurity. Curr Opin Ophthalmol 2003;14(5): 286–90.
115. Phelps DL. Retinopathy of prematurity. Curr Probl Pediatr 1992;22(8):349–71.
116. Cryotherapy for Retinopathy of Prematurity Cooperative Group. Multicenter trial of cryotherapy for retinopathy of prematurity. Three-month outcome. Arch Ophthalmol 1990;108(2):195–204.
117. Cryotherapy for Retinopathy of Prematurity Cooperative Group. Multicenter trial of cryotherapy for retinopathy of prematurity: one-year outcome—structure and function. Arch Ophthalmol 1990;108(10):1408–16.
118. Cryotherapy for Retinopathy of Prematurity Cooperative Group. Multicenter Trial of Cryotherapy for Retinopathy of Prematurity: ophthalmological outcomes at 10 years. Arch Ophthalmol 2001;119(8):1110–8.
119. Higgins R. Retinopathy of prematurity. E-Medicine 2006. Available at: www.emedicine.com/ped/topic1998.htm. Accessed March 25, 2007.
120. Ng EY, Connolly BP, McNamara JA, et al. A comparison of laser photocoagulation with cryotherapy for threshold retinopathy of prematurity at 10 years: part 1. Visual function and structural outcome. Ophthalmology 2002;109(5):928–34.
121. Connolly BP, Ng EY, McNamara JA, et al. A comparison of laser photocoagulation with cryotherapy for threshold retinopathy of prematurity at 10 years: part 2. Refractive outcome. Ophthalmology 2002;109(5):936–41.
122. Paysse EA, Lindsey JL, Coats DK, et al. Therapeutic outcomes of cryotherapy versus transpupillary diode laser photocoagulation for threshold retinopathy of prematurity. J AAPOS 1999;3(4):234–40.

123. Hunter DG, Repka MX. Diode laser photocoagulation for threshold retinopathy of prematurity. A randomized study. Ophthalmology 1993;100(2):238–44.
124. Laser ROP Study Group. Laser therapy for retinopathy of prematurity. Arch Ophthalmol 1994;112:154–6.
125. Ling CS, Fleck BW, Wright E, et al. Diode laser treatment for retinopathy of prematurity: structural and functional outcome. Br J Ophthalmol 1995;79:637–41.
126. White JE, Repka MX. Randomized comparison of diode laser photocoagulation versus cryotherapy for threshold retinopathy of prematurity: 3-year outcome. J Pediatr Ophthalmol Strabismus 1997;34:83–7.
127. Shalev B, Farr AK, Repka MX. Randomized comparison of diode laser photocoagulation versus cryotherapy for threshold retinopathy of prematurity: seven-year outcome. Am J Ophthalmol 2001;132:76–80.
128. Andersen CC, Phelps DL. Peripheral retinal ablation for threshold retinopathy of prematurity in preterm infants. Cochrane Database Syst Rev 2000;(2):CD001693.
129. Phelps DL, Retinopathy of prematurity: a practical clinical approach. Neo Reviews 2001;2(7):e174–9
130. McNamara JA. Laser treatment for retinopathy of prematurity. Curr Opin Ophthalmol 1993;4:76–80.
131. Topilow HW, Ackerman AL. Cryotherapy for stage 3+ retinopathy of prematurity: visual and anatomic results. Ophthalmic Surg 1989;20(12):864–71.
132. Noorily SW, Small K, de Juan E Jr, et al. Scleral buckling surgery for stage 4B retinopathy of prematurity. Ophthalmology 1992;99:263–8.
133. Trese MT. Scleral buckling for retinopathy of prematurity. Ophthalmology 1994;101:23–6.
134. Hinz BJ, deJuan E Jr, Repka MX. Scleral buckling surgery for active stage 4A retinopathy of prematurity. Ophthalmology 1998;105:1827–30.
135. Hubbard GB III, Cherwick DH, Burian G. Lens-sparing vitrectomy for stage 4 retinopathy of prematurity. Ophthalmology 2004;111:2274–7.
136. Lakhanpal RR, Sun RL, Albini TA, et al. Anatomic success rate after 3-port lens-sparing vitrectomy in stage 4A or 4B retinopathy of prematurity. Ophthalmology 2005;112:1569–73.
137. Prenner JL, Capone A Jr, Trese MT. Visual outcomes after lens sparing vitrectomy for stage 4A retinopathy of prematurity. Ophthalmology 2004;111:2271–3.
138. Repka MX, Tung B, Good WV, et al. Outcome of eyes developing retinal detachment during the Early Treatment for Retinopathy of Prematurity Study (ETROP). Arch Ophthalmol 2006;124(1):24–30.
139. Sears JE, Sonnie C. Anatomic success of lens-sparing vitrectomy with and without scleral buckle for stage 4 retinopathy of prematurity. Am J Ophthalmol 2007;143(5):810–3.
140. Ferrone PJ, Harrison C, Trese MT. Lens clarity after lens-sparing vitrectomy in a pediatric population. Ophthalmology 1997;104:273–8.
141. Lakhanpal RR, Davis GH, Sun RL, et al. Lens clarity after threeport lens-sparing vitrectomy in stage 4A and 4B retinal detachments secondary to retinopathy of prematurity. Arch Ophthalmol 2006;124(1):20–3.
142. Hartnett ME. Features associated with surgical outcome in patients with stages 4 and 5 retinopathy of prematurity. Retina 2003;23(3):322–9.

143. Spaide RF, Fisher YL. Intravitreal bevacizumab (Avastin) treatment of proliferative diabetic retinopathy complicated by vitreous hemorrhage. Retina 2006;26: 275–8.
144. Avery RL, Pieramici DJ, Rabena MD, et al. Intravitreal bevacizumab (Avastin) for neovascular age-related macular degeneration. Ophthalmology 2006;113: 363e5–72e5.
145. Chung EJ, Kim JH, Ahn HS, et al. Combination of laser photocoagulation and intravitreal bevacizumab (Avastin) for aggressive zone I retinopathy of prematurity. Graefes Arch Clin Exp Ophthalmol 2007;245:1727–30.
146. Shah PK, Narendran V, Tawansy KA, et al. Intravitreal bevacizumab (Avastin) for post laser anterior segment ischemia in aggressive posterior retinopathy of prematurity. Indian J Ophthalmol 2007;55:75–6.
147. Travassos A, Teixeira S, Ferreira P, et al. Intravitreal bevacizumab in aggressive posterior retinopathy of prematurity. Ophthalmic Surg Lasers Imaging 2007;38: 233–7.
148. Cryotherapy for Retinopathy of Prematurity Cooperative Group. Multicenter trial of cryotherapy for retinopathy of prematurity. Snellen visual acuity and structural outcome at 5 1/2 years after randomisation. Arch Ophthalmol 1996;114:417–42.
149. Ruth A, Hutchinson AK, Hubbard GB III. Late vitreous hemorrhage in patients with regressed retinopathy of prematurity. J AAPOS 2008;12:181–5.
150. Tasman W, Brown GC. Progressive visual loss in adults with retinopathy of prematurity (ROP). Trans Am Ophthalmol Soc 1988;86:367–79.
151. Cats BP, Tan KE. Prematures with and without regressed retinopathy of prematurity: comparison of long-term (6–10 years) ophthalmological morbidity. J Pediatr Ophthalmol Strabismus 1989;26(6):271–5.
152. Cryotherapy for Retinopathy of Prematurity Cooperative Group. Multicenter trial of cryotherapy for retinopathy of prematurity: natural history ROP: ocular outcome at 5(1/2) years in premature infants with birth weights less than 1251 g. Arch Ophthalmol 2002;120(5):595–9.

# The Ten Commandments of Pain Assessment and Management in Preterm Neonates

Marlene Walden, PhD, APRN, NNP-BC, CCNS[a,*], Carol Carrier, MSN, RN, CNS[b]

**KEYWORDS**

• Pain • Neonate • Assessment • Management • Preterm

The last three decades have brought about tremendous change in the way that care providers view and treat pain in the preterm neonate. Long ago, the myth that preterm infants do not feel pain because of the immaturity of their central nervous system provided rationale for lack of treatment. One only has to spend a short time observing preterm neonates during procedures in the Neonatal Intensive Care Unit (NICU) to know that preterm infants do indeed feel pain. Despite impressive gains in the scientific evidence related to the assessment and management of pain in neonates, treatment decisions and implementation of evidence-based practice ultimately falls to the doctors and other health care practitioners who provide care for these vulnerable patients on a day-to-day basis. Families expect that their infant in the NICU is receiving special attention to the prevention and management of pain. They rarely question practitioners because they assume their infant's pain is being managed appropriately.

The case study that follows is probably one of the most poignant examples of the gap that still exists between research and implementation of scientific evidence into routine clinical practice. This article presents the Ten Commandments of pain assessment and management in the NICU from a preterm infant's point of view for the consideration of practitioners and nurses who advocate for and strive to provide compassionate neonatal care.

[a] School of Nursing, The University of Texas, 1700 Red River, Mailcode D0100, Austin, TX 78701–1499, USA

[b] Newborn Center, Texas Children's Hospital, AB 480, 6621 Fannin Street, Houston, TX 77030, USA

* Corresponding author. School of Nursing, The University of Texas, 1700 Red River, Mailcode D0100, Austin, TX 78701–1499.

*E-mail address:* mwaldennnp@aol.com (M. Walden).

Crit Care Nurs Clin N Am 21 (2009) 235–252
doi:10.1016/j.ccell.2009.02.001 ccnursing.theclinics.com

## CASE STUDY OF A 23-WEEK-OLD PRETERM NEONATE

"I work in a level III neonatal intensive care unit. We care for many extremely preterm infants, some as young as 22- to 23-weeks of gestation, weighing under a pound. We recently had an infant who was just 23 weeks. Due to a large patent ductus arteriosus (PDA), she was given indomethacin and required a second course because the ductus did not close. She was briefly on a high-frequency ventilator. She developed necrotizing enterocolitis (NEC) and was taken to the operating room (OR) for an ileostomy (all this at less than a pound). During all this, she began to lose her skin and began to third space. Candida was found in the section of bowel that was removed. She was given amphotericin, vancomycin, and claforan. She had no urine output, and was taken back to the OR for a PDA ligation. Her blood urea nitrogen (BUN) was 67 and creatinine 2.0. She was in septic shock and disseminating intravascular coagulation. They were pouring blood and platelets into her. She was blown up like a balloon. Venous access was near impossible, so they decided to place a Broviac catheter at the time of the ligation. Keep in mind with all this going on, NO PAIN MEDICATION WAS GIVEN. The thoracic surgeon would not do the ligation due to the condition of the infant, but the pediatric surgeon did agree to place the Broviac. There had been no urine output for three days and no blood pressure in 24 hours. Dopamine was started. She survived the Broviac placement. Still no pain medication. Skin was coming off in sheets and she was bleeding from many areas on the body. Her right ear was necrotic, and the abdominal incision was oozing pus and opening up due to the third spacing. They finally agreed to prescribe morphine every 3 to 4 hours PRN ("as needed"). NONE of the nurses caring for the child would give it because the baby did NOT appear to be in pain! I finally convinced one nurse to give the morphine and she felt bad about giving it because the baby showed no sign of pain. She went another 10 hours before I pushed for the nurse to give it again. At the time of the baby's death she was still receiving only occasional doses of morphine. BUN was 79, creatinine 4, no urine output in 7 days, overwhelming sepsis, and her heart finally gave out."[1]

## CASE STUDY DISCUSSION

In this case study, the preterm neonate was experiencing acute, disease-related pain. Infants who have NEC[2] often require analgesia when their abdomens distend and become extremely tender to touch. This infant was subjected to multiple painful procedures and surgical interventions with minimal pharmacologic pain relief. There is no information about her environment; it is optimistic to presume that developmental support was in place for this infant.

Following surgery that results in an ileostomy, a postoperative pain management plan in anticipation of pain is expected. A Broviac catheter for central access was later placed without analgesia. Only after her status continued to deteriorate from overwhelming infection was morphine prescribed PRN. Sadly, PRN medications commonly are not given as frequently as scheduled pain medications. It is important to recognize that infants near death are often incapable of demonstrating clear pain responses, because there is little energy for motor arousal and movement or even facial expressions to indicate the need for pain intervention. Even though many of her nurses probably considered giving an analgesic, they were torn between preconceived notions that impaired their ability to see the reality of the situation, and the need to provide ongoing relief at end of life for this neonate.

Despite the despair engendered while evaluating this case, there is optimism that increasing numbers of caregivers aspire to improve neonatal pain assessment and management. It is our hope that these Ten Commandments provide the impetus for practitioners and staff to improve pain assessment and management in the NICU.

## THE TEN COMMANDMENTS

### *1. Take Time to Consider Whether You Can Prevent Me From Experiencing Pain As Part of My Medical Care*

The first commandment centers around the belief that the best way to prevent pain is to avoid causing it in the first place. To fully implement this commandment, practitioners ought to examine the way they provide care in the NICU. Except on rare occasions, clinical procedures should be scheduled on an as-needed basis versus a routine schedule.[3] Each laboratory or diagnostic test should be evaluated for medical necessity and how the information gained might be used to potentially alter the infant's plan of care. If no action will be taken on the results obtained, the practitioner should carefully consider whether the laboratory or diagnostic test is needed. If the test is determined to be necessary, the grouping of laboratory and diagnostic procedures should be evaluated to reduce infant exposure to increasing numbers of painful procedures. For example, routine laboratory tests can be drawn at the same time as a time-sensitive test (ie, antibiotic drug level) instead of exposing the infant to multiple separate painful procedures. In addition, noninvasive monitoring devices may be used whenever possible to guide medical interventions, thereby limiting the number of laboratory tests needed.[3] If frequent laboratory tests are unavoidable, the practitioner should consider establishing central venous/arterial access to minimize skin-breaking procedures. In terms of other pain-reducing strategies, the practitioner should use minimal amounts of tape/adhesives and consider using skin barrier products when possible to prevent injury and pain upon removal.

Painful procedures performed at the same time as other nonemergency routine care (eg, taking vital signs, changing a diaper) may result in sensory hypersensitivity (referred to as the "wind-up phenomenon"), causing non-noxious stimuli to be perceived as painful.[4] Furthermore, handling and immobilization in preparation for painful procedures may heighten activity in nociceptive pathways and accentuate the infant's pain responses, and therefore should be minimized.

In summary, it is important to prevent or minimize pain whenever possible by reducing the number of painful procedures performed on infants. It is also essential to properly premedicate before invasive procedures every single time to ensure prevention of pain and later consequences of unrelieved repetitive painful events.

### *2. My Signs of Pain May Be Subtle or Brief, But It Does Not Mean That I Don't Have Pain*

Although pain responses in preterm neonates may be subtle, brief, or nonexistent, it is important to remember that what is painful to an adult or child is also painful to a preterm infant, regardless of their ability to communicate the pain. Presently, no easily administered, widely accepted, uniform technique exists for assessing pain in infants. A multidimensional pain assessment tool that includes measurements for both physiologic and behavioral indicators of pain is preferable, given the multifaceted nature of pain. In addition, caregivers should select instruments with tested reliability, validity, and clinical utility. Infant population, setting, and type of pain experienced should also guide selection of a pain instrument.[5] The four most commonly used multidimensional infant-specific pain assessment tools with psychometric data include the Premature Infant Pain Profile (PIPP),[6] the CRIES neonatal pain assessment tool,[7] the Neonatal Infant Pain Scale (NIPS),[8] and the Neonatal Pain, Agitation, and Sedation Scale (N-PASS).[9]

The PIPP (**Table 1**) was originally developed to measure procedural pain,[6] but recently has also been used in term and preterm infants to assess postoperative pain.[10,11] While the PIPP may be presumed to be valid only with preterm neonates, the instrument has been tested in neonates ranging from extremely preterm to 40 weeks' postconceptional age. The PIPP incorporates two contextual factors that may account for an infant's less robust pain responses that may result from their immaturity or behavioral state. By scoring infants who are younger or those who are asleep higher on the PIPP, the adjusted scores do not penalize infants who are known to be less capable of mounting a robust response to noxious stimuli. The PIPP contains two physiologic indicators (ie, heart rate and oxygen saturation) and three facial indicators (ie, brow bulge, eye squeeze, and nasolabial furrow). While total scores vary between 18 and 21, depending on the infant's gestational age, scores between 7 and12 usually signify mild-to-moderate pain requiring nonpharmacologic comfort measures and scores greater than 12 indicate moderate-to-severe pain requiring pharmacologic pain intervention in addition to comfort measures.[6]

The CRIES (**Table 2**) is another instrument that has been used extensively to assess pain in the newborn.[7] Originally developed to assess postoperative pain in infants 32 to 36 weeks' gestational age, recent studies have documented its clinical utility in assessing procedural pain in preterm and term neonates.[12–14] CRIES is an acronym for the five parameters it measures: Crying, Requires increased oxygen administration, Increased vital signs, Expression, and Sleeplessness. Total scores for the CRIES range from 0 to10, with scores less than four indicative of mild pain requiring nonpharmacologic pain relief measures and scores greater than or equal to five consistent with moderate-to-severe pain requiring pharmacologic intervention in conjunction with comfort measures.[7]

The NIPS (**Table 3**), like the PIPP, was originally developed to assess procedural pain in preterm and term newborns,[8] but recent literature also validates its use with postoperative pain.[15,16] The NIPS examines five behavioral parameters (ie, facial expression, crying, arms, legs, and state of arousal) and one physiologic parameter (ie, breathing pattern). Total score ranges from zero to seven. Scoring of the NIPS does not contain physiologic parameters requiring cardiorespiratory monitoring, thus it is particularly useful in assessing pain in healthy, term infants. Although guidelines for pain interventions based on total score are not provided by NIPS researchers, all pain instruments in neonates are based on the premise of increasing pain intensity. Therefore, when using tools without scoring guidelines for pain management, when an infant's pain scores reach the midrange of the total possible points for that tool (ie, approximately four or greater with the NIPS), the practitioner may accurately infer that the infant is experiencing moderate-to-severe pain, and that pharmacologic intervention for that pain is warranted.

The N-PASS (**Table 4**) measures both pain/agitation and sedation in preterm and term neonates who have prolonged pain postoperatively and during mechanical ventilation.[9] The five-item N-PASS contains four behavioral items (crying/irritability, behavior state, facial expression, extremities/tone) and one physiologic indicator (vital signs). Like the PIPP, points are added to the preterm neonate's pain score based on their gestational age to compensate for their limited ability to behaviorally or physiologically communicate pain. Total pain scores vary depending on the infant's gestational age, but scores greater than three usually signify pain requiring nonpharmacologic comfort measures and/or pharmacologic pain intervention. The sedation portion of the N-PASS requires an assessment of response to stimuli and can be useful in titrating opioid requirements based on level of sedation desired. Sedation is scored between 0 and −2 for each behavioral and physiologic criterion, then summed and noted as a negative score (0 to −10). Scores of −10 to −5 is considered deep sedation, while light sedation scores range from −5 to −2.

### *3. Take the Time to Manage My Pain Appropriately and Put My Needs Ahead of Your Own*

The third commandment is a poignant reminder to remember the Golden Rule. "Do unto others as you would have them do unto you" is probably the single greatest, simplest, and most important moral adage ever invented, one that appears in the writings of almost every culture and religion throughout history. In terms of pain management in preterm neonates, this commandment reminds us to examine our motives and uncover what drives our pain management choices. Practitioners and staff often allow busy clinical schedules to drive the choice not to use analgesia for painful procedures because of the added time involved. Instead of being honest with themselves, they may attribute the infant's pain response to other aspects of caregiving. For example, a common myth that is often heard regarding circumcision is that the infant was crying in response to being strapped down on the circumcision board versus crying in response to the painful surgical removal of the foreskin covering the glans of the penis. Practitioners need to take responsibility for their choices instead of hiding behind excuses. If the practitioner is in doubt that the infant is in pain, the default should always be to give the infant the benefit of the doubt and at least consider a trial of analgesic therapy.

The long-term impact of a change in philosophy by caregivers in terms of ensuring proper premedication before invasive procedures becomes readily apparent when considering the vast number of painful procedures that a preterm infant in the NICU is routinely subjected to. Carbajal and colleagues[17] found that infants born between 24 and 42 weeks' gestation experienced a mean of 98 painful procedures during the first 14 days of admission, with one neonate having 364 painful procedures. Many of the procedures commonly performed in the neonate cause moderate-to-severe pain, with average pain scores of five on a 10-point scale.[18] Substantial numbers of failed attempts at procedures dramatically increase the number of painful procedures that neonates are subjected to. In that same study, some of the most painful procedures needed as many as 10 to 15 attempts for completion. These frequent, invasive, and noxious procedures occur randomly in the NICU and often are not routinely managed with either pharmacologic or nonpharmacologic interventions.[17,18] For individual caregivers, the accumulation of an infant's painful procedures is not noticeable as we come and go on our job schedules, so missing analgesia for "just this one procedure" may be deceptive when compared with the actual occurrence of painful events during an infant's hospital stay.

### *4. Stay with Me During Painful Procedures to Help Me Cope with the Pain and Stress—Your Presence and Gentle Hands Give Me Strength*

Painful procedures in the NICU are unavoidable; therefore it is vital that caregivers assist infants to cope with and recover from medically necessary, painful clinical procedures. Positioning and containment strategies have been investigated as nonpharmacologic strategies to minimize pain in the neonatal population. A hand-swaddling technique known as "facilitated tucking" (holding the infant's extremities flexed and contained close to the trunk), has been shown to reduce pain responses in preterm neonates. In a study by Corff and colleagues,[19] preterm infants who were hand-swaddled in this manner before undergoing a heelstick procedure demonstrated significantly reduced heart rates and crying, and more stability in sleep–wake cycles. Hand-swaddling was also demonstrated to be effective in reducing procedural pain of

**Table 1**
**Premature infant pain profile (PIPP)**

| Process | Indicator | 0 | 1 | 2 | 3 | Score |
|---|---|---|---|---|---|---|
| Chart | Gestational age (weeks) | ≥36 | ≥32–<36 | ≥28–<32 | <28 | — |
| Score 15 seconds immediately before event | Behavioral state | Active/awake<br>Eyes open<br>Facial movements | Quiet/awake<br>Eyes open<br>No facial movements | Active/sleep<br>Eyes closed<br>Facial movements | Quiet/sleep<br>Eyes closed<br>No facial movements | — |
| Record baseline heart rate ___ Observe infant 30 seconds immediately following event | Maximum heart rate | 0–4 beats/ minute increase | 5–14 beats/ minute increase | 15–24 beats/ minute increase | ≥25 beats/ minute increase | — |
| Record baseline oxygen sat. ___ Observe infant 30 seconds immediately following event | Minimum oxygen saturation | 0 to 2.4% decrease | 2.5% to 4.9% decrease | 5.0% to 7.4% decrease | ≥7.5% decrease | — |

| | | | | | | |
|---|---|---|---|---|---|---|
| Observe infant 30 seconds immediately following event | Brow bulge | None 0% to 9% of time | Minimum 10% to 39% of time | Moderate 40% to 69% of time | Maximum ≥70% of time | — |
| Observe infant 30 seconds immediately following event | Eye squeeze | None 0% to 9% of time | Minimum 10% to 39% of time | Moderate 40% to 69% of time | Maximum ≥70% of time | — |
| Observe infant 30 seconds immediately following event | Nasolabial furrow | None 0 to 9% of time | Minimum 10% to 39% of time | Moderate 40% to 69% of time | Maximum ≥70% of time | — |
| — | — | — | — | — | Total | Score ____ |

*From* Stevens B, Johnston C, Petryshen P, & Taddio A. Premature infant pain profile: development and initial validation. Clinical Journal of Pain 1996;(12):13–22; with permission.

**Table 2**
**CRIES: neonatal postoperative pain assessment score**

| Indicator | 0 | 1 | 2 |
|---|---|---|---|
| Crying | No | High-pitched | Inconsolable |
| Requires $O_2$ for saturation >95% | No | <30% | >30% |
| Increased vital signs | Heart rate and blood pressure within 10% of preoperative value | Heart rate and blood pressure 11% to 20% higher than preoperative value | Heart rate and blood pressure 21% or more above preoperative value |
| Expression | None | Grimace | Grimace/grunt |
| Sleeplessness | No | Wakes at frequent intervals | Constantly awake |

*From* Krechel S, Bildner J. CRIES: A new neonatal postoperative pain measurement score: initial testing of validity and reliability. Pediatric Anesthesia1995;5(1): 53–61; with permission.

**Table 3**
**Neonatal infant pain scale (NIPS)**

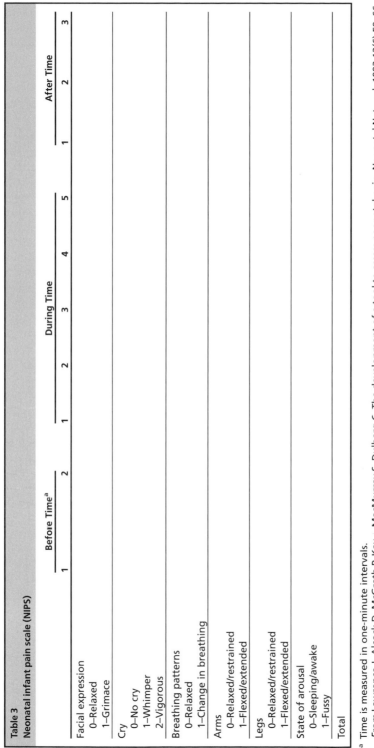

| | Before Time[a] | | During Time | | | | | After Time | | |
|---|---|---|---|---|---|---|---|---|---|---|
| | 1 | 2 | 1 | 2 | 3 | 4 | 5 | 1 | 2 | 3 |
| Facial expression<br>0–Relaxed<br>1–Grimace | | | | | | | | | | |
| Cry<br>0–No cry<br>1–Whimper<br>2–Vigorous | | | | | | | | | | |
| Breathing patterns<br>0–Relaxed<br>1–Change in breathing | | | | | | | | | | |
| Arms<br>0–Relaxed/restrained<br>1–Flexed/extended | | | | | | | | | | |
| Legs<br>0–Relaxed/restrained<br>1–Flexed/extended | | | | | | | | | | |
| State of arousal<br>0–Sleeping/awake<br>1–Fussy | | | | | | | | | | |
| Total | | | | | | | | | | |

[a] Time is measured in one-minute intervals.

*From* Lawrence J, Alcock D, McGrath P, Kay J, MacMurray S, Dulberg C. The development of a tool to assess neonatal pain. Neonatal Network 1993;12(6):59–66, with permission.

**Table 4**
**Neonatal pain, agitation, and sedation scale**

| | Sedation | | Normal | Pain/Agitation | |
|---|---|---|---|---|---|
| **Assessment Criteria** | -2 | -1 | 0 | 1 | 2 |
| Crying Irritability | No cry with painful stimuli | Moans or cries minimally with painful stimuli | Appropriate crying<br>Not irritable | Irritable or crying at intervals<br>Consolable | High-pitched or silent continuous cry<br>Inconsolable |
| Behavior State | No arousal to any stimuli<br>No spontaneous movement | Arouses minimally to stimuli<br>Little spontaneous movement | Appropriate for gestational age | Restless, squirming<br>Awakens frequently | Arching, kicking<br>Constantly awake or arouses minimally/no movement (not sedated) |
| Facial Expression | Mouth is lax<br>No expression | Minimal expression with stimuli | Relaxed Appropriate | Any pain expression, intermittent | Any pain expression, continual |
| Extremities Tone | No grasp reflex<br>Flaccid tone | Weak grasp reflex muscle tone | Relaxed hands and feet<br>Normal tone | Intermittent clenched toes, fists, or finger splay<br>Body is not tense | Continual clenched toes, fists, or finger splay<br>Body is tense |
| Vital Signs HR, RR, BP, $SaO_2$ | No variability with stimuli<br>Hypoventilation or apnea | <10% variability from baseline with stimuli | Within baseline or normal for gestational age | 10%–20% from baseline $SaO_2$ 76%–85% with stimulation-quick | > 20% from baseline $SaO_2$ <75% with stimulation-slow, out of sync with vent |

*Notes:* (1) Pain and sedation scores are recorded separately. (2) Points are added to the premature infant's pain score based on their gestational age: + 3 if < 28 weeks' gestation/corrected age; + 2 if 28–31 weeks' gestation/corrected age; + 1 if 32–35 weeks gestation/corrected age. (3) Sedation assessment requires an assessment of response to stimuli.

*From* Hummel P, Puchalski M, Creech SD, et al. Clinical reliability and validity of the N-PASS: neonatal pain, agitation, and sedation scale with prolonged pain. J Perinatol 2008;28(1):55–60, with permission.

endotracheal suctioning.[20] There is also evidence that supports parents as effective providers of facilitated tucking during painful procedures with their preterm infants.[21]

A similar containment study conducted by Fearon and colleagues[22] used blanket swaddling for nesting. The researchers examined the effectiveness of blanket swaddling after a heelstick in younger (less than 31 weeks' postconceptual age) and older (at or older than 31 weeks' postconceptual age) preterm infants. Trends showed that blanket swaddling was effective for reducing heart rate and negative facial displays in the post-heelstick phase for the older infants and increased oxygen saturation levels in younger infants.

Skin-to-skin contact during painful procedures reduces pain scores (PIPP), facial expression, crying, and heart rate in preterm newborns and neonates.[23,24] Skin-to-skin or "kangaroo care" holding is another option for parents who are comfortable with the procedure and want to participate in comforting their infant during painful procedures.

Pacifiers have longed been used as a nonpharmacologic strategy for pain in the NICU. Pacifiers offer the opportunity for the infant to engage in nonnutritive sucking, which is hypothesized to modulate transmission or processing of nociception through mediation by the endogenous nonopioid system. The efficacy of nonnutritive sucking is immediate, but appears to terminate almost instantly upon cessation of sucking.

Pain relief is greater in infants who receive both nonnutritive sucking and sucrose. Studies demonstrate that a single 0.05 to 2 mL dose of 0.24 to 0.50 g (12% to 25%) sucrose given orally approximately 2 minutes before painful stimulus is associated with statistically and clinically significant reductions in crying after a painful stimulus. Sucrose is hypothesized to modulate transmission or processing of nociception through the release of endogenous opioids triggered by the sweet taste of sucrose.[25] The safety of implementing repeated doses of sucrose in extremely preterm neonates has not been confirmed; therefore caution is advised before widespread use of repeated doses in this population.[3] However, in a study by Stevens and colleagues,[26] no immediate adverse effects were noted when administering a 24% sucrose-dipped pacifier during four random, consecutively administered, routine heelstick procedures.

Lastly, environmental modifications such as reduced lighting and noise levels help to minimize infant stress during caregiving procedures, and are especially important following painful episodes so that infants can recover without an ongoing source of stressful stimuli.

### *5. Use Best Pharmacologic Practices to Manage My Pain My Life Rests in Your Hands*

Pharmacologic agents are often required to alleviate moderate-to-severe procedural, postoperative, or disease-related pain in neonates.[27] Intravenous opioids remain the most common class of analgesics administered in the NICU, particularly that of morphine sulfate and fentanyl citrate.

Morphine can be administered either as a bolus dose (0.05 to 0.2 mg/kg/dose by IV slow push, intramuscularly, or subcutaneous route every 4 hours) or as a continuous infusion (give loading dose of 0.1 to 0.15 mg/kg over 1 hour followed by a continuous infusion of 0.01 to 0.02 mg/kg/hour). The onset of action begins a few minutes after IV administration, with peak analgesia occurring at 20 minutes.[28]

The effectiveness of morphine for acute pain caused by invasive procedures remains unclear. Although earlier studies supported the effectiveness of morphine analgesia for acute pain,[29–31] more recent studies refute its effectiveness.[32] No analgesic efficacy of intravenously administered morphine was noted on endotracheal tube suctioning or heelsticks.[33,34]

Fentanyl has a more rapid onset and shorter duration of action compared with morphine and must be administered as a continuous infusion (1 to 5 mcg/kg/hour) or as an intravenous bolus (1 to 4 mcg/kg/dose every 2 to 4 hours by slow IV push). The onset is almost immediately after IV administration.[28] Fentanyl offers two distinct advantages over morphine. First, fentanyl causes less histamine release than morphine and may be more appropriate for infants who have hypovolemia or hemodynamic instability, congenital heart disease, or ex-preterm infants who have chronic lung disease.[35] Secondly, fentanyl blunts increases in pulmonary vascular resistance. This finding makes it potentially useful in managing pain in neonates who have persistent pulmonary hypertension, in neonates during extracorporeal membrane oxygenation, and in neonates following cardiac surgery.[35]

Whether morphine or fentanyl is used for pain management, the efficacy of opioid therapy should be assessed using a valid and reliable neonatal pain scale. Sedation level should also be assessed regularly, monitoring for the attainment of desired sedation level or inadvertent oversedation.

Acetaminophen is a nonsteroidal anti-inflammatory drug commonly used for short-term use with mild-to-moderate pain in neonates.[28] For oral dosing, administer a 20 to 25 mg/kg loading dose followed by a maintenance dose of 12 to15 mg/kg/dose. The loading dose for rectal administration is 30 mg/kg followed by a maintenance dose of 12 to 18 mg/kg/dose. Maintenance intervals vary by gestational age and are recommended every 6 hours for term infants, every 8 hours for preterm infants greater or equal to 32 weeks, and every 12 hours for preterm infants younger than 32 weeks.[28] Adverse effects of acetaminophen include liver toxicity, rash, fever, thrombocytopenia, leukopenia, and neutropenia.

EMLA cream (eutectic mixture of lidocaine and prilocaine, local anesthetics) is the most widely studied topical anesthetic in neonates and is approved in infants at birth with a gestational age of 37 weeks or greater. EMLA cream reduces pain during venipuncture, circumcisions, arterial puncture, and percutaneous venous catheter placement, but is not effective for management of pain associated with the heelstick procedure.[36] The topical dose is 1 to 2 g under occlusive dressing 60 to 90 minutes before procedure.[28] Adverse effects include methemoglobinemia, redness, and blanching.

Liposomal lidocaine cream (LMX 4%; Ferndale Laboratories, Michigan) is a relatively new topical anesthetic for use in newborns. LMX may be a better choice than EMLA because of its faster onset of action and no risk of methemoglobinemia.[37] However, further studies in neonates are needed to establish the safety and efficacy of LMX for management of procedural pain in neonates.

### *6. Make Sure You Know the Side Effects of Pain Medications and Monitor Me Closely to Keep Me Safe—I Place My Trust in You*

Morphine has few effects on the neonatal cardiovascular system in the well-hydrated neonate. Hypotension, bradycardia, and flushing are part of the histamine response to morphine and can be decreased by slow intravenous bolus administration (over 10 to 20 minutes) and optimizing intravascular fluid volume.[35,38] As morphine predisposes patients to hypotension, a recent study by Hall and colleagues[39] recommends that morphine administration in preterm neonates between 23 and 26 weeks with preexisting hypotension be used with caution because morphine has been found to be associated with adverse neurologic outcomes including severe intraventricular hemorrhage and death.

Although relatively uncommon, the effects of histamine release may also cause bronchospasm in infants who have chronic lung disease.[35] Enterohepatic recirculation of morphine may contribute to rebound increases in plasma levels and late respiratory depression.[40,41]

Decreased intestinal motility and abdominal distention may also occur, causing a delay in the establishment of enteral feeding in preterm neonates.[42] The effect of morphine on gastrointestinal motility is hypothesized to be dose-dependent, and tolerance of enteral feeds may be improved by priming the gut with small volumes of milk and lower doses of morphine.[35]

Rarely, fentanyl can significantly reduce chest wall compliance (stiff chest syndrome). This naloxone-reversible side effect can be prevented by slow infusion (as opposed to rapid bolus administration), administration of doses less than 3 mcg/kg, or concomitant use of muscle relaxants.

The administration of fentanyl is associated with a modest increase in intracranial pressure. Caution is therefore recommended for administration of fentanyl to patients with intracranial pathology.[35]

Increased intraabdominal pressure can triple the elimination half-life of fentanyl, probably because of reduced hepatic artery blood flow. Although it has only been demonstrated for fentanyl, increased intraabdominal pressure probably occurs with other opioids that are metabolized by the liver. Because many neonates experience increased intraabdominal pressure, elimination is an important consideration in administering opioids to neonates.[35]

Because opioids may in some instances be administered concurrently with adjunctive agents, it is important to remember that sedatives suppress the behavioral expression of pain and have no analgesic effects. Sedatives should only be used when pain has been ruled out. When administered with opioids, sedatives may allow more optimal weaning of opioids in critically ill, ventilator-dependent neonates who have developed tolerance from prolonged opioid therapy. The two most commonly used sedatives in neonates include midazolam and chloral hydrate. However, no research has been done to determine the safety or efficacy of combining sedatives and analgesics for the treatment of pain in infants.

Finally, a word of caution about using neuromuscular blocking agents. Chemical paralysis is often used for severely ill neonates. Because the use of paralytic agents masks the behavior signs of agitation or pain, sedatives or analgesics should be used in conjunction with paralytics.

### *7. Be Aware That However You Manage My Pain, I Will Never Forget It*

Repetitive, unrelieved pain can lead to serious and adverse consequences for neonates. Short-term physiologic consequences of painful procedures include decreased oxygen saturations and increased heart rates that can place increased demands on the cardiorespiratory system. Pain can cause elevation in intracranial pressure, thereby increasing risk of intraventricular hemorrhage in preterm neonates. Pain and stress may also depress the immune system and contribute to increased susceptibility of neonates to infections.

The long-term effects of pain in animals are clear, with changes observed in pain thresholds, social behaviors, stress responses, and pain responses to nonpainful stimuli.[43] Preliminary human data suggest that early pain experiences may alter future pain responses. Johnston and Stevens[44] reported that neonates who were born at 28 weeks' gestation and were hospitalized in an NICU for 4 weeks (32 weeks' postconceptional age) had decreased behavioral response and significantly higher heart and lower oxygen saturation during a heelstick procedure compared with newly born neonates at 32 weeks' gestation. In another study, Taddio and colleagues[45] reported that males circumcised within 2 days of birth had significantly longer crying bouts and higher pain intensity scores at immunization at 4 or 6 months of age than males who were not circumcised.

### *8. Please Take Care When You Discontinue or Wean My Pain Medications Because I May Have Become Dependent On These Medications and Need You to Monitor My Vital Signs and Behaviors For Signs of Opioid Withdrawal*

Neonates who require opioid therapy for more than several days should be weaned slowly to prevent withdrawal symptoms such as signs of neurologic excitability, gastrointestinal dysfunction, autonomic signs, poor weight gain, and skin excoriation due to excessive rubbing. The prevalence of opioid withdrawal is greater in infants who have received fentanyl as opposed to morphine. Similarly, infants who receive higher total doses or longer duration of infusion are significantly more likely to experience withdrawal.[46] Data are insufficient to determine the optimal weaning rate of opioids to prevent withdrawal symptoms in neonates on opioid therapy. Ducharme and colleagues[47] reported that adverse withdrawal symptoms in children who received continuous infusions of opioids and/or benzodiazepines could be prevented when the daily rate of weaning did not exceed 20% for children who received opioids/benzodiazepines for 1 to 3 days, 13% to 20% for 4 to 7 days, 8% to 13% for 8 to 14 days, 8% for 15 to 21 days, and 2% to 4% for more than 21 days. An opioid weaning scale such as the Finnegan Scoring System assists in the management of opioid withdrawal in neonates exposed to prolonged opioid therapy.[48]

### *9. Include My Parents and Other Caregivers in Decisions That Affect My Care—It Is Crucial For My Well-Being*

Parents have many concerns and fears about their infant's pain and about the medications used in the treatment of pain.[49,50] Parents may fear the effects of pain on their child's development. They may also fear that their infant may become "addicted" to the analgesics.[51] Parents and health care professionals must talk openly and honestly about acute and chronic pain associated with medical diseases, and about pain associated with operative, diagnostic, and therapeutic procedures. Practitioners should provide parents with accurate and unbiased information about the risks and benefits of (and alternatives to) analgesia and anesthesia, so that they can make informed treatment choices.[52] When determining the infant's pain management plan, the parents' cultural and religious beliefs about pain should be taken into consideration. Lastly, parents can learn how their infant expresses pain through physiologic and behavioral cues and how they can assist caregivers in providing nonpharmacologic pain relief during minor painful procedures that their infant experiences.

### *10. If and When My Death Draws Near, Please Stay With Me and My Parents—Everything Is Easier If You Are There to Comfort and Care For Me and My Family*

Practitioners in the NICU may regularly experience moral distress that arises from competing interests to support dying infants with advanced technology when palliative or comfort care would be more humane. Practitioners also may feel unprepared to respond adequately to the emotional devastation of parents and other family members.[53] In response, practitioners may develop varying coping strategies to manage these morally distressing situations, including focusing on the physical care of the dying infant rather than on the emotional and spiritual support of the infant and family. Ongoing professional support from colleagues and professional organizations are available to help practitioners cope with these extremely difficult situations so that they can in turn provide the needed emotional support to a dying infant and their family.

Assessment of pain presents special challenges at end of life because dying infants may be too ill to exhibit behavioral signs of pain, thus rendering neonatal pain tools largely ineffective. Therefore, caregivers must often consider risk factors for pain and rely on physiologic measures such as increases in heart rate and decreases in oxygen saturation to make pain management decisions.

Pain management at end of life primarily centers on the provision of opioids to minimize pain and nonpharmacologic therapies to enhance the infant's comfort level.[54] Continuous infusions of opioid therapy such as morphine and fentanyl are often required to manage pain at end of life and should be titrated to desired clinical response (analgesia).[35] Opioid dosages well beyond those described for standard analgesia are often required for infants who are in severe pain or who have developed tolerance (decreasing pain relief with the same dosage over time) after the prolonged use of opioids.[55] Although caregivers may be concerned about the appearance of hastening death in the dying neonate, the risk of hastening death is not an appropriate reason to withhold adequate analgesia.[56] In addition to pharmacologic interventions, physiologic comfort measures may palliate pain and distressing symptoms in infants at end of life and include reduction of noxious stimuli, organization of caregiving, and positioning and containment strategies.[53] A high priority during palliative and comfort care is that parents are given many opportunities to nurture, provide care, and comfort their infant. Appropriate pain management is one tool that helps accomplish this goal.

## SUMMARY

Despite advances in pain assessment and management, nonpharmacologic and pharmacologic analgesic therapies continue to be underutilized to manage both acute and procedural pain in preterm neonates. Untreated acute, recurrent, or chronic pain related to disease or medical care may have significant and lifelong physiologic and psychological consequences. Painful procedures in the NICU may be unavoidable, so it is vital that caregivers balance the painful, but medically necessary care with evidence-based nonpharmacologic and pharmacologic strategies to relieve pain and stress. Practitioners can use the Ten Commandments as a reminder to relieve suffering whenever possible as a nursing and ethical commitment to infants and families. By following the guiding principle of "Do unto others' infants as you would want them to do for your own," practitioners and staff will, we hope, be motivated to provide the compassionate care that these tiny, vulnerable preterm infants need and deserve.

## REFERENCES

1. Anand KJS, Rovnagh C, Walden M, et al. Consciousness, behavior and clinical impact of the definition of pain. Pain Forum 1999;8:64–73.
2. Gibbins S, Maddalena P, Moulsdale W, et al. Pain assessment and pharmacologic management for infants with NEC: a retrospective chart audit. Neonatal Netw 2006;25(5):339–45.
3. Walden M, Gibbins S, editors. Pain assessment and management: guideline for practice. 2nd edition. Glenview (IL): National Association of Neonatal Nurses; 2008. p. 1–29.
4. Holsti L, Grunau RE, Oberlander TF, et al. Prior pain induces heightened motor responses during clustered care in preterm infants in the NICU. Early Hum Dev 2005;81(3):293–302.
5. Duhn LJ, Medves JM. A systematic integrative review of infant pain assessment tools. Adv Neonatal Care 2004;4(3):126–40.

6. Stevens B, Johnston C, Petryshen P, et al. Premature Infant Pain Profile: development and initial validation. Clin J Pain 1996;12(1):13–22.
7. Bildner J, Krechel SW. Increasing staff nurse awareness of postoperative pain management in the NICU. Neonatal Netw 1996;15(1):11–6.
8. Lawrence J, Alcock D, McGrath P, et al. The development of a tool to assess neonatal pain. Neonatal Netw 1993;12(6):59–66.
9. Hummel P, Puchalski M, Creech SD, et al. Clinical reliability and validity of the N-PASS: neonatal pain, agitation and sedation scale with prolonged pain. J Perinatol 2008;28(1):55–60.
10. McNair C, Ballantyne M, Dionne K, et al. Postoperative pain assessment in the neonatal intensive care unit. Arch Dis Child Fetal Neonatal Ed 2004;89(6): F537–41.
11. El Sayed MF, Taddio A, Fallah S, et al. Safety profile of morphine following surgery in neonates. J Perinatol 2007;27(7):444–7.
12. Ahn Y. The relationship between behavioral states and pain responses to various NICU procedures in premature infants. J Trop Pediatr 2006;52(3):201–5.
13. Belda S, Pallas CR, De la Cruz J, et al. Screening for retinopathy of prematurity: is it painful? Biol Neonate 2004;86(3):195–200.
14. Herrington CJ, Olomu IN, Geller SM. Salivary cortisol as indicators of pain in preterm infants: a pilot study. Clin Nurs Res 2004;13(1):53–68.
15. Rouss K, Gerber A, Albisetti M, et al. Long-term subcutaneous morphine administration after surgery in newborns. J Perinat Med 2007;35(1):79–81.
16. Suraseranivongse S, Kaosaard R, Intakong P, et al. A comparison of postoperative pain scales in neonates. Br J Anaesth 2006;97(4):540–4.
17. Carbajal R, Rousset A, Danan C, et al. Epidemiology and treatment of painful procedures in neonates in intensive care units. JAMA 2008;300(1):60–70.
18. Simons SH, van Dijk M, Anand KS, et al. Do we still hurt newborn babies? A prospective study of procedural pain and analgesia in neonates. Arch Pediatr Adolesc Med 2003;157(11):1058–64.
19. Corff KE, Seideman R, Venkataraman PS, et al. Facilitated tucking: a nonpharmacologic comfort measure for pain in preterm neonates. J Obstet Gynecol Neonatal Nurs 1995;24(2):143–7.
20. Ward-Larson C, Horn RA, Gosnell F. The efficacy of facilitated tucking for relieving procedural pain of endotracheal suctioning in very low birthweight infants. MCN Am J Matern Child Nurs 2004;29(3):151–6 [quiz 157–8].
21. Axelin A, Salantera S, Lehtonen L. 'Facilitated tucking by parents' in pain management of preterm infants-a randomized crossover trial. Early Hum Dev 2006;82(4):241–7.
22. Fearon I, Kisilevsky BS, Hains SM, et al. Swaddling after heel lance: age-specific effects on behavioral recovery in preterm infants. J Dev Behav Pediatr 1997; 18(4):222–32.
23. Castral TC, Warnock F, Leite AM, et al. The effects of skin-to-skin contact during acute pain in preterm newborns. Eur J Pain 2008;12(4):464–71.
24. Johnston CC, Stevens B, Pinelli J, et al. Kangaroo care is effective in diminishing pain response in preterm neonates. Arch Pediatr Adolesc Med 2003;157(11): 1084–8.
25. Anseloni VC, Ren K, Dubner R, et al. A brainstem substrate for analgesia elicited by intraoral sucrose. Neuroscience 2005;133(1):231–43.
26. Stevens B, Johnston C, Franck L, et al. The efficacy of developmentally sensitive interventions and sucrose for relieving procedural pain in very low birth weight neonates. Nurs Res 1999;48(1):35–43.

27. Golianu B, Krane E, Seybold J, et al. Non-pharmacological techniques for pain management in neonates. Semin Perinatol 2007;31(5):318–22.
28. Young TE, Mangum B. NeoFax: a manual of drugs used in neonatal care. 20th edition. Montvale (NJ): Thomson Healthcare; 2007.
29. Anand KJ, Barton BA, McIntosh N, et al. Analgesia and sedation in preterm neonates who require ventilatory support: results from the NOPAIN trial. Neonatal Outcome and Prolonged Analgesia in Neonates. Arch Pediatr Adolesc Med 1999; 153(4):331–8.
30. McCulloch KM, Ji SA, Raju TN. Skin blood flow changes during routine nursery procedures. Early Hum Dev 1995;41(2):147–56.
31. Scott CS, Riggs KW, Ling EW, et al. Morphine pharmacokinetics and pain assessment in premature newborns. J Pediatr 1999;135(4):423–9.
32. Anand KJ, Johnston CC, Oberlander TF, et al. Analgesia and local anesthesia during invasive procedures in the neonate. Clin Ther 2005;27(6):844–76.
33. Carbajal R, Lenclen R, Jugie M, et al. Morphine does not provide adequate analgesia for acute procedural pain among preterm neonates. Pediatrics 2005; 115(6):1494–500.
34. Simons SH, van Dijk M, van Lingen RA, et al. Routine morphine infusion in preterm newborns who received ventilatory support: a randomized controlled trial. JAMA 2003;290(18):2419–27.
35. Anand KJS, Menon G, Narsinghani U, et al. Systemic analgesic therapy. In: Anand KJS, Stevens BJ, McGrath PJ, editors. Pain in neonates. 2nd edition. Amsterdam: Elsevier Science; 2000. p. 159–88.
36. Taddio A, Ohlsson A, Einarson TR, et al. A systematic review of lidocaine-prilocaine cream (EMLA) in the treatment of acute pain in neonates. Pediatrics 1998;101(2):E1–9.
37. Lehr VT, Cepeda E, Frattarelli DA, et al. Lidocaine 4% cream compared with lidocaine 2.5% and prilocaine 2.5% or dorsal penile block for circumcision. Am J Perinatol 2005;22(5):231–7.
38. Stoelting R. Handbook of pharmacology & physiology in anesthetic practice. Philadelphia: Lippincott, Williams.Wilkins; 1995.
39. Hall RW, Kronsberg SS, Barton BA, et al. Morphine, hypotension, and adverse outcomes among preterm neonates: who's to blame? Secondary results from the NEOPAIN trial. Pediatrics 2005;115(5):1351–9.
40. Bhat R, Abu-Harb M, Chari G, et al. Morphine metabolism in acutely ill preterm newborn infants. J Pediatr 1992;120(5):795–9.
41. Bhat R, Chari G, Gulati A, et al. Pharmacokinetics of a single dose of morphine in preterm infants during the first week of life. J Pediatr 1990;117(3):477–81.
42. Saarenmaa E, Huttunen P, Leppaluoto J, et al. Advantages of fentanyl over morphine in analgesia for ventilated newborn infants after birth: a randomized trial. J Pediatr 1999;134(2):144–50.
43. Goldschneider KR, Anand KS. Long-term consequences of pain in neonates. In: Schechter NL, Berde CB, Yaster M, editors. Pain in infants, children, and adolescents. 2nd edition. Philadelphia: Lippincott Williams & Wilkins; 2003. p. 58–70.
44. Johnston CC, Stevens BJ. Experience in a neonatal intensive care unit affects pain response. Pediatrics 1996;98(5):925–30.
45. Taddio A, Goldbach M, Ipp M, et al. Effect of neonatal circumcision on pain responses during vaccination in boys. Lancet 1995;345(8945):291–2.
46. Dominguez KD, Lomako DM, Katz RW, et al. Opioid withdrawal in critically ill neonates. Ann Pharmacother 2003;37(4):473–7.

47. Ducharme C, Carnevale FA, Clermont MS, et al. A prospective study of adverse reactions to the weaning of opioids and benzodiazepines among critically ill children. Intensive Crit Care Nurs 2005;21(3):179–86.
48. Finnegan LP, Kron RE, Connoughton JF, et al. A scoring system for evaluation and treatment of the neonatal abstinence syndrome: a new clinical and research tool. In: Morselli PI, Garatani S, Sereni F, editors. Basic and therapeutic aspects of perinatal pharmacology. New York: Raven Press; 1975. p. 139–53.
49. Gale G, Franck LS, Kools S, et al. Parents' perceptions of their infant's pain experience in the NICU. Int J Nurs Stud 2004;41(1):51–8.
50. Franck LS, Allen A, Cox S, et al. Parents' views about infant pain in neonatal intensive care. Clin J Pain 2005;21(2):133–9.
51. Franck LS, Cox S, Allen A, et al. Parental concern and distress about infant pain. Arch Dis Child Fetal Neonatal Ed 2004;89(1):F71–5.
52. Harrison H. The principles for family-centered neonatal care. Pediatrics 1993; 92(5):643–50.
53. Rogers S, Babgi A, Gomez C. Educational interventions in end-of-life care: part I: an educational intervention responding to the moral distress of NICU nurses provided by an ethics consultation team. Adv Neonatal Care 2008;8(1):56–65.
54. Walden M, Sudia-Robinson T, Carrier CT. Comfort care for infants in the neonatal intensive care unit at end of life. Newborn Infant Nurs Rev 2001;1(2):97–105.
55. Partridge JC, Wall SN. Analgesia for dying infants whose life support is withdrawn or withheld. Pediatrics 1997;99(1):76–9.
56. Gale G, Brooks A. Implementing a palliative care program in a newborn intensive care unit. Adv Neonatal Care 2006;6(1):37–53.

# Living with Grief Following Removal of Infant Life Support: Parents' Perspectives

Debra Armentrout, RN, NNP, PhD

**KEYWORDS**

- Neonatal death • Perinatal loss
- Removal of neonatal life support • Grounded theory

Birth generally is regarded as a time of joy and hope. It is a time for dreaming about the future and celebrating the continuity of life. Babies are expected to be born healthy, without any sign of illness. When a newborn infant dies, the family's hopes and dreams die as well. Ongoing advances in neonatology and modern technology have reduced neonatal morbidity and mortality significantly. Despite the marvels of modern neonatal intensive care practices, however, infant death remains a reality, and questions frequently are raised about whether continued treatment of a critically ill infant is futile and possibly inhumane.

Approximately 34,000 neonatal deaths occur annually in the United States,[1] many of which occur after removal of life support. Formerly the decision to continue or stop the use of life support measures for a critically ill infant was made primarily by physicians; now, parents are now encouraged to participate in the decision. The thought of losing a newborn infant is incomprehensible to most parents, and participating in making the decision about life support for their infant verges on the surreal.[2]

Research findings reported in the literature about making life and death decisions for critically ill infants in the neonatal ICU (NICU) focus primarily on the experiences of health care providers and the ethical dilemmas surrounding these decisions. Fewer studies focus on parents' experiences in making decisions about discontinuing life support for the infant, and even fewer address what life is like for parents following the death of the infants. Therefore the author conducted a qualitative study as part of her doctoral requirements that explored with parents how life support decisions were made for their infants, the roles they had in the decision-making process, and how the decisions and subsequent deaths of their infants influence their everyday lives. The results of that qualitative investigation, *Holding a Place: A Grounded Theory of Parents Bringing Their Infant Forward in Their Daily Lives Following the Removal of*

Clinical Pediatrics, University of Texas Medical School, 6431 Fannin Street, Houston, TX 77030, USA

*E-mail address:* debra.c.armentrout@uth.tmc.edu

Crit Care Nurs Clin N Am 21 (2009) 253–265

doi:10.1016/j.ccell.2009.01.003

ccnursing.theclinics.com

*Life Support and Subsequent Infant Death*, have been described elsewhere.[3,4] This article expands on the concepts identified by parents as factors in their decision making and on the facilitators and barriers the parents faced, and continue to face, in their grieving process.

## SAMPLE

After approval from the institutional review boards of the sponsoring universities, participants were recruited from a large support group for parents who experienced the neonatal death of a child. Recruitment material that described the study's purposes was published in the support group's on-line newsletter accessed electronically via the group's Web site. The theoretical sample for this study was comprised of 15 parents, four couples and seven mothers whose spouses chose not to participate. Interviews were conducted either face-to-face or via telephone.

Most participants (13) were white; one was Hispanic, and one was African American. Thirteen participants identified themselves as being of Christian faith, one had vowed to raise the child as a Jew, and one was self-described as being spiritual. The educational levels of the participants ranged from a year of college to a master's degree. Annual household incomes ranged from \$50,000 to \$100,000. Study participants ranged in age from 27 to 42 years (mean = 31.6 years) at the time of the infant's death. The time that had elapsed between the death of the infant and the participation of the parents in this study ranged from 0.5 to 12 years (mean = 3.9 years).

All losses discussed during the study were single losses (one child). In two cases of twin births, the one surviving twin in each pair was alive and well. The gestational ages of the infants ranged from 25 to 41 weeks. Three infants had lethal congenital defects, two were extremely premature, two had congenital heart defects (CHD), one had lethal pulmonary disease, one had early-onset sepsis, one experienced hypoxic-ischemic encephalopathy, and for one infant the cause of death remained unknown. Ten of the infants ranged in age from 2 to 12 days at the time that the decision to remove life support was made. The decision for one infant was made at 2 months of age during a re-hospitalization for emergency heart surgery.

Following the decision to remove life support, nine of the infants died within minutes (range = 2–40 minutes) to hours (range = 1–6 hours). Two infants died at home, one at 14 and one at 40 days of age. Two participants reported having had one previous perinatal loss from miscarriage, eight participants had other children living at the time of their neonate's death, and six participants reported they had a child or children born to them after the death of their neonate.[3,4]

## DATA COLLECTION

Data in this grounded theory study were narrative interviews. Each participant was asked the same opening question: "Tell me about your son/your daughter." Parents then were asked to describe what it was like to realize that their infant was not going to survive. Parents were asked to describe what their lives were like immediately after their infant's death and how their lives are now, without the infant. Parents also were asked about their current feelings regarding their decisions and if, in retrospect, they would do anything differently. Participants were encouraged to share their thoughts and memories of the infant, what the infant's brief presence in their lives meant to them, and how the decisions they made influenced the ways their lives have evolved. Either during or at the end of each interview, parents were asked what advice they have for parents currently involved in facing such a decision. Finally, each participant was asked what he or she believed was important to share about their experiences that had not been addressed.[2,3]

**MAKING THE DECISION**

All participants spoke of the dawning realization that, despite hope and prayer, their infant was not going to survive. One parent stated that "the decision was pretty clear cut … He wasn't going to get better," whereas another commented that "there wasn't a big decision … There wasn't any need to go on … He was just suffering, and we didn't want him to suffer." Some parents perceived their infant to be "slowly dying, so if we did not remove the life support, he would die on his own;" others felt the infant "was just artificially kept alive, and I don't think he was really there." Although making the decision to remove the infant from life support was described as "heartbreaking," "a nightmare of a situation … just a horror … just a very painful thing," the parents interviewed felt that not withdrawing support would be a "selfish thing to do," "something to satisfy my empty arms." Deciding to remove their infant from life support was expressed as "the hardest decision we've ever had to make" but, considering "the magnitude of what the baby was going through," also "the most loving" decision the parent could make for the child.

Having to process the harsh reality of their infant's impending death, parents perceived that they "did the best we could under the circumstances." "If there had been hope … a chance for a cure … a full recovery or even a somewhat normal life existence, though difficult, that would be different," but "in our hearts we knew there was nothing more, and it was the best decision." Another mother touchingly stated, "I would do everything … well, we felt like we did … we exhausted all that we could, and this was what was best for her."

Having made the decision to remove the infant from life support allowed parents "more private time" with their infant as a family. For some it was their only opportunity to hold and talk to their infant like "a normal baby without all the tubes and wires." A mother of a premature infant with oligohydramnios recognized that her daughter "would have left the world with all the tubes, and that's just not something that I wanted. … I would have had to live with that for a long time, too. I think this was better. She got to hear her dad sing, she got to … she knew we were holding her so … yeah, I think we made the best decision. I have doubts, like I said, about if she would have fought for another day … but I don't have the regrets. It's hard to imagine what your life would have be like if you would have made another decision. There would have been a lot of images I would have had to live with. … It would have been a different way for her to go. It wouldn't have been holding her. … It would have been sitting there … looking at her … on the bed." Similar feelings were expressed by a mother of an infant failing to come off extracorporeal membrane oxygenation when she tearfully explained, "They asked me if I wanted to, like, pull the tubes out completely—that would require another surgery—or just clamp them off and cut them. And I was afraid that with another surgery he would already be dead when I would get to hold him, so we just clamped them. We stayed there for a little while, and we carried him back to that room. …We were alone then." This ability to hold the infant as death occurred created a bittersweet memory that was described by all participants. One mother summed up this sentiment for all parents in the study when she voiced that "holding her when she died … that's not a memory I want to have to have, but … my feeling is, if your child has to die, what better place than in mom's arms … so … I try and make that a good memory, but it's a very sad good."

## THINGS THEY WOULD HAVE CHANGED

Believing that "there was nothing that anybody could do to make it better ... your baby's going to die," the parents in this study did not express any guilt over their decision to remove their critically ill infant from life support and continue to believe that it "was the right thing to do" under the circumstances. They did, however, express some regrets about how they spent the time they shared with the infant after making the decision. These regrets centered primarily on three different areas: (1) parenting acts not performed ("I didn't look at her hair, you know, to see how much hair she had, I didn't take the time to look at her body and just study every little bit of her." "Personally my only regret was that I didn't bathe him ... that day and that I didn't dress him ... in the outfit that I wanted to see him in."), (2) taking pictures and creating other memories ("We took a lot of pictures ... but I don't think you ever have enough." "The nurses did a little foot plaster of her feet, and then they cut it out of the shape of a heart, a little bow on it ... and I'll tell you what ... that was awesome having that was just ... one of the most special things." "And the baptism ... why didn't we do it sooner ... why did we wait for somebody on call to show up with a bottle of sterile water and a cotton ball ...why didn't we do it the right way?"), and (3) having friends and family see and know their infant ("I think later it would have helped with our grief to have had more family involvement in the hospital experience." "I would have invited more people to see her before ... we took her off life support ... because to me the more people that would have seen her ... they would have realized our loss more." "The only thing we might have done ... some of our closest friends ... it would have been nice to have them there as well ... none of our friends got to see or meet him while he was alive.") These activities would have contributed to future memories and provided testimony to their infant's brief existence.

When asked what advice they had for other couples facing a similar decision, study participants frequently identified activities housed within these three areas such as "clipping his hair, his fingerprints, his footprints ... have pictures with him ... we never had a family portrait with him." One father of a premature daughter said, "You have to cherish every minute that you have with them." One mother commented that she tells other families to "take that time with their baby ... to hold their hand and to really love them and care about them. I think it's important to allow yourself to be a mother before you let go ... of the baby ... to be a parent to some degree ... to change their diaper ... feed 'em if you can ... play with their toes and fingers and nose and ... just be a mother to 'em ... be a parent to 'em ... before you turn it off, because that ... is something that you will cherish for the rest of your life." Families that were able to take their babies home commented, "It was an easier time. ... People could come and go as they pleased" and "I wanted them to spend time with her, hold her, and bathe her and do whatever." One mother explained that having her infant son at home for a period of time "made it more personable, because you could actually have true memories with your house." Despite this period being one of the "toughest times" of their lives, being able to have their infant with them as part of a family was something that all parents proclaimed they "would never replace for anything in the world."

An area of uncertain regret for those participants who had other living children at the time of the infant's death was whether they should have involved the baby's siblings differently. One mother, already the mother of three children, commented that she "might have had my kids there more than I did ... and I even recently I considered ... should I have had my older children with us when we took her off life support? ... I don't know the answer, but I've considered thinking I wonder if we should have said do you want to be with us ... should we have included them more ... would it have made it easier for them … I don't know." Similarly, the mother of four previous children and a twin to the deceased infant, stated "that the day that we went to remove her from life support … that morning we explained to the kids what her situation was, and that we didn't know for sure if she would be coming back, and we would be taking pictures. … We had already been taking pictures, but what I did was I got a tape recorder, and I had all the kids record … introduce themselves on the tape recorder, and we, we played that for her at the hospital … but the social worker was encouraging us to let the kids come, but … it was so painful. … We didn't want them to feel what we were feeling, … but, like I said, now I know they were feeling pain … that is one thing I wish I could have changed."

**HEALTH CARE PROVIDERS**

Most of the study participants' experiences with health care professionals were of a positive nature. One father of a premature son reflected that "the nursing staff, the doctors … they really know what they're doing … not only medically, but dealing with us personally … that helped a lot." The parents deeply appreciated actions acknowledging the infant as a person in his or own right before the death. The mother of a daughter who had congenital anomalies remarked that "one of the nurses wrote down that she liked to be swaddled … and that she didn't like it when her diapers were wet. … It was like a piece of information … that gave me something about her character." "Calling in on their days off to see how he was doing … requesting to be assigned to him" showed parents that their infant mattered to others.

Study participants also valued health care professionals' support and empathy for the horrific situation the participants faced. One mother expressed that she perceived it as "such a great blessing … that there was no hindrance in the terms of any kind of an attitude or anything with the nurse or the attending doctor that made us feel uncomfortable or gave us any additional grief." Several parents expressed appreciation for the tears shed by health care providers for their infant, because "it meant so much to know that others were sad" for their infant, "that he was more than just another patient."

When asked how health care professionals could have helped more during this extremely emotional period, parents responded "to encourage them to be parents … during that time … help them to collect memories … pictures as a family … hair cuttings … plaster feet … blankets … sound kind of unimportant … but mean so much." It was later in their grieving that parents occasionally commented that health care professionals "dropped the ball." As a mother of a son who had CHD describes, "the medical professionals who have become your support system and your family while your child was alive … all of a sudden they're gone … I think it's important to have some kind of support system or information … otherwise it's like stepping into this huge abyss." In asking what advice she would have for health care professionals, another mother sighed as she commented that she "would want them to know that it lasts … the grief lasts longer than they will ever imagine … that it affects families on a deeper level than they will ever imagine … that what happens in the NICU … that families carry that with them forever."

**INITIAL SHOCK**

Mothers repeatedly commented that, despite performing normal activities, they were essentially dysfunctional for lengthy periods of time. One mother of a term infant stated that she would "would get up in the morning … I would be … normal … after about 2 weeks, 3 weeks … act normally … take the little one to school, stay in the car for a while … come back home and get into bed for the next 6 hours … and cry, and do whatever I needed to do ... and I'd say, "OK gotta go get her, so I guess I'd better shower." You know, get up, take a shower, get dressed, go pick her up ... then it was little baby steps. I would go home, and I wouldn't get into bed, I would sit on the sofa. I have a very leafy backyard, and I would sit on the sofa and stare ... just stare. I was incredulous for a very long time. I was just in shock for a very long time. The milestone of a year was really bad. And it is still bad. I mean I'm functioning. I put on make-up. I get dressed. I go out. I look normal ... but it lasts for along time ... the bad thing." Another mother who lost a daughter to hypoxic-ischemic encephalopathy felt her son "was the only thing I felt I had to get up for in the morning ... but I guess I feel like I lost about a year of my son's time. He turned 3 shortly after my daughter died, and it wasn't ... until he was a little after 4 that I turned around in the kitchen and saw this little boy ... and said 'Who are you?" ... I wasn't all there for about a year ... and this little boy, even though he was the one who got me through it ... I really didn't know who he was." Another mother who lost a son to group B streptococcal sepsis commented that she believed it to be "time, more time ... I was nonfunctional for the first year. ... For the first couple of months I could hardly leave the house. ... It was like leaving the house was like a sensory overload. I had so much energy going into coping I couldn't do anything else. ... Parenting my surviving child took every ounce of energy that I had. ... The first year was just awful. ... The second year was not a lot better, but I was pregnant again, and so I had that to focus on but ... it was probably 3 years before I could really ... I really felt I had turned a milestone."

The fathers in the sample commented that "although we're hurting every day, we get up and continue on." Undertaking household projects and returning to work was described by fathers in the study as their "grief work." One father's description of those initial days following the death of his son was that "your mind is always on it ... regardless of how busy you are. ... There are always reminders ... no matter where you turn. ... You just have to realize ... that you're not doing yourself any justice or your child any justice. ... You'll be doing them a bigger disservice by not attempting to get on with your life ... not being able to do the everyday tasks that everybody else has to do. ... You have to get up. ...You have to ... get back in the grind. ...You have to go back to work. ... You can't just ... life ... can't stop. ... Life just doesn't stand still. ... It has to keep going ... in order for people to survive and in order for memories to carry on. ... You have to ... keep functioning."

In asking what advice they would give to other couples grieving in a similar situation, study participants uniformly commented that there "wasn't a set formula" and that people had to "allow themselves to feel sad ...to feel bad." That, unfortunately, one should "try not to avoid the pain. ... The more you try to put it behind you or rise above it or whatever ... you just can't ... you're just gonna have to go through that agony. ... There's just no way out of it." As one mother explained "people kind of give you a year to be absent minded and kind of ditzy, but after that you should be OK. And that's just not the case. ... That hasn't been my experience."

Parents interviewed all suggested "not to expect too much of yourself for a long time" and "not to let anybody push you into doing or going or being or acting how they think you should be. ... You deal with it with what works for you." "If that's just a little for you, well, then, it's a little for you. ... But if you're really wanting to grieve a lot, and everyone's telling you it's sufficient, you just need to listen to your own heart."

## DIFFERENCES IN GRIEF BETWEEN MOTHERS AND FATHERS

Some parents had been informed that differences in grieving would occur between couples that had lost an infant; others were not provided with this information. One mother who lost a daughter to a lethal congenital anomaly stated that being provided this information "helped save our marriage" because her husband "wasn't on the same page with me, and it almost seemed like a betrayal." Although all couples commented that it was important for them "to stick together … with your spouse … and make decisions together and communicate together and … and no matter what it takes … you've lost enough with losing a baby, … and you don't need to lose your marriage, so … just stick together and talk and communicate," this communication and shared grieving occurred primarily in the days before and immediately after their infants' death. "We grieved … while our son was alive, we really clung to each other … for the immediate aftermath. I can't think back and not feel his arms around me. … I mean, he was terribly supportive, and … then, I would say after about 5 or 6 months, the only thing we had in common was that we had lost the same child. … Everything was different." Mothers found themselves "needing to talk," to "just to sit and cry," to "research the Internet," to "visit the cemetery every day," to "send flowers," whereas fathers "alphabetized the garage, changed all the doorknobs in the house," "did something physical, hit balls at batting cages." One father of a premature infant explained that "I did a lot of crying around the time he died and up until the point he died, even, but … basically, from the funeral on, … as much as it hurt, that just didn't happen for me so … it was hard for me to understand sometimes why she was … and it was hard for me to figure out OK what am I suppose to do … but … I don't think I ever resented the fact that we've grieved differently. … I think I've become more understanding," to which his wife responded, "I came to realize pretty quickly that his grief was just different from mine. … He wasn't crying on the outside … like I was 24/7, which I didn't understand how he could not be … but he definitely was on the inside. … I think we pretty quickly figured out that we were just responding in different ways." For them it was a matter of "just respecting each other's differences." One mother commented that although her husband "definitely went through his grieving a lot more quickly than I did, he never made me feel like I wasn't allowed to grieve, and anytime I wanted to talk about it, he pretty much would stop what he was doing and give me his full attention … allow me to talk." Another mother who had lost her son 12 years before the interview, however, commented that she would ask her husband "to talk. … You know, I said, 'Tell me what this is like … you have to share with me,' but it's never been his thing. … Then every once in awhile he … 1 year he surprised me, and he had written a poem … and 1 year he bought a star … you know, the star registry, … and last year he shows up, it was a surprise, he had taken our son's footprints … and he had a tattoo put on his upper arm of his footprints … so you know I know that it's still there for him … but he just, he doesn't talk about it very much." For another mother it was necessary "to give each other space. … It's a long, hard process, but … if you stick together, … everything will be worth it in the end." Although parents interviewed acknowledged the differences in the way they demonstrated their grief, one mother quietly sighed as she said, "It's been 6 years, and I know he grieves. … I still just wish he grieved the way I do."

### FAMILY AND FRIENDS

Many parents had very supportive families and friends, but others found themselves facing further hurt when people close to them did not recognize their loss. Parents frequently commented that "the reality that there was a child and a life that came and went seemed to have been lost on a lot of people" and that "not treating her as if she was a person that was here … is hurtful." As one parent responded back to family members who viewed another family member's stillbirth at 4 months as more of a "real loss" than the death of his 25-week daughter at 3 days of age, "No, we had our hopes and dreams shattered right before our eyes. Once you hold a child, regardless of their size, there's a lot of things going through your mind. You're thinking about for their future and all the fun times you're going to share as a family and all that." His wife added, "She was here. She … held your hand. My dad took his ring and slipped it up her arm. She was a person that was here." One mother with a surviving twin commented how hurtful it was when family members did not attend her deceased infant's funeral, "almost like the baby was not a significant family member." Another parent expressed that "people just think, 'Oh, the baby died.' … Well, you know they didn't see her, it doesn't mean so much."

Parents interviewed felt that friends and family "wanted to be helpful and supportive, but people didn't know what to say." As one mother stated, "I think the things they were saying were suppose to be right and helpful … but they didn't feel right and helpful." One mother was told "'But you have three other beautiful children …,' and I say 'But I had four.'" One father was frequently told "'Oh, you'll get through this, you'll have another baby'… I mean, this is such an experience … that the last thing you want to think about is having kids." One mother, on being told that she can always have anther baby, tearfully responded "But it wouldn't be that baby." Parents frequently were told "At least you didn't have her long enough to miss her," that the baby "is in a better place," that it "was part of God's plan," or "at least you didn't bring her home," remarks they described as "hurtful." One parent suggested that people "felt like they needed to say something positive, and they felt like I needed to put a positive spin on something that doesn't have one."

What parents identified as being helpful from friends and family "was just "being there … for us … that is what we needed. … If we wanted to cry, they were there for that. … If we wanted to just throw an anger fit, they were there for that." Having friends and family that "didn't overwhelm us … they just let us tell them what we needed, and they would respond. … They would basically just let us know they were just there for uz, that they cared … was a lot more important and effective in helping us deal with our grief." One father commented that "communicating your feelings to somebody that you trust was probably the thing that gets me through almost on a daily basis."

## FEELINGS OF ISOLATION

Having the support of family and friends for the horrific decision they had to make "was important not … just our recovery … coming through grief … but knowing they supported our decision and supported us … made the process easier than … it would have been otherwise." Several of the study participants, however, revealed that they have "never really told outside friends or distant families that we actually took him off the ventilator. … I didn't think it was anyone's business … except our families." In searching for information on infant loss, one mother discovered not finding anything "about having to make the decision to take your child off life support. … I think it's probably something that people don't want to talk about." Even participation in a parent loss support group was difficult, as the mother of a daughter who had congenital heart disease explained, "This is not something that you normally hear … people who have had similar experiences taking them off life support." Although none of the parents expressed regret over their decision to remove life support, parents felt that they would like the opportunity to "kind of compare … issues … and feelings," and "to talk to somebody who has been through it and has survived." A mother of four older children and a surviving twin sibling to a daughter born with lethal congenital defects echoed this sentiment as she poignantly commented she does "not have the opportunity to talk with parents that have had babies on life support and had to remove them. … And I just kind of wanted to know what other parents think"

## REMEMBERING ACTIVITIES

Study participants identified several strategies for remembering their infant that helped them with their grief and loss over time. Most mothers put together a memory box or scrapbook containing the few "tangible things I have of her … which I share with her siblings, family, … just everyone." Every day one mother wears "an angel of some sort … and that's what it's for … that's how I remember her." Another mother wears "the little necklace that has your children's charms on it, … and I wear five of them." Special Christmas ornaments are "bought every year and hung with the other kids' ornaments … and they know those are his." A father of an infant who had congenial anomalies frequently stops by the cemetery where his son is buried: "I talk out loud … about my day … what's going on. … Talking to him now … because he's not here … that's what helps … I guess keeps me grounded." One mother involves herself in various causes "because of her … like the Heart Walk, … and for her 1-year birthday I ran a blood drive; … just anything I think of that … I would have done only because she was here … and I needed to help." One mother whose infant was cremated "planted a garden in the front yard … bought a special fountain for next to her stone … made her seem more permanent."

## MOVING FORWARD

With the passage of time parents realized that they had to "move on. … Life will never be the same …. You'll be forever changed, … but you do have to go on with your life. … You have to find a new normal for you." A mother of a premature son stated that for her it was that "all of a sudden I realized it's okay that I don't cry every day. … I still cry, but I think you have to realize that there's still joy in life. … Yes, we lost a son, but life is still … the sun still comes up, and there are still good things in the world, and there are still things to look forward to." Even though they have moved forward, there is still a void that never goes away. One mother commented, "There's just a hole that will never get filled up … not with another baby, … not with anything. … I mean, there's just no filling that hole. It's just always there. … Sometimes its closer to the surface, and other times it's not, but it never goes away. … It just never goes away." One mother compared her loss of 12 years earlier to "people who lose limbs … there's never a day they don't wish their arm or leg was there, but they learn to function in spite of its absence, and I think losing a child is very much like that … when there's always an awareness that someone is not there that should be there, but … you learn to function in spite of it." Another mother who had an infant who had CHD 6 years earlier views "losing a baby like back pain … you injured your back, it's never going to be the same, … and you get used to … there are certain things you can and can't do with your injury, … and it's always there, … but it's lightened up a lot, … but it's never going to go away. … It's the same thing with my grief. … It's there. … I can just deal with it now, … and I know there are just some things I can't do, … and there's some things I can do. … You know, … but it's an injury, so to speak, that's just always going to be there, … and you just … have to accept that it's always going to be there, … and you, you work around it. … I think most people think grief is something that's going to go away, … and I don't, I don't agree. … Maybe there are certain griefs that do, but not grief over losing a child. … It doesn't go away. …You learn how to handle it, that's all. … That's not an easy thing to learn how to do."

Essential to study participants' ability to move forward was their belief that their infant was still "very much a part of our family, even though she's not here." This belief was verified by one mother who proclaimed, "She is not left out because she's dead, and I think because of that we go forward, and we're OK." Another mother explained, "She's here, but I guess in a different way. We've just incorporated her into our lives in a different way than the other kids. … That's been important to us." A poignant example of maintaining her infant's presence in the family was illustrated by one of the mothers when she commented, "We have her pictures up with everybody else's. … Everybody else gets a new picture every year for school, except hers is the same. … But that's just the way it is. … Every now and then I come across … well, I don't come across—we only have about 2 dozen photos of her to begin with … I'll think, 'Maybe that one we can turn and crop, and do this, and do that and make it a new one,' and that's really exciting when I manage how to do that."

All parents described maintaining an awareness of the deceased infant for both older and subsequent siblings. One mother commented, "He's our son, he always will be. … Our daughter points to his picture. … She knows that's her brother, and she will always know that that's her brother, and he may not be here with us physically, but he's always going to be a part of our lives." Another mother, in sharing how she maintains an awareness of her deceased infant with her children, described that she "always had photos of him up. … His footprints are framed and also hanging up. … I have a hope chest with his belongings from the hospital and stuff from the pregnancy, the blankie, and … his urn, and those kinds of things that I've shared with them. … I went ahead and put together a baby book for him, and I've shared that with them." A mother who commented, "On his birthday we go to the beach. Of course, when they were little, my other children didn't understand the significance, but as they grew older and were able to … they now know that that's where his ashes are scattered" provided another example of including siblings.

## ALTERED PERSPECTIVES OF LIFE

All study participants talked about a shift in life priorities as they emerged from their intense grief and loss. "It kind of re-focuses you. … There are some things in life that really matter, and there are other things that just don't." As one mother explained, "Things that used to seem like a big deal just aren't a big deal. My perspective has changed a little bit. I hope I'm more compassionate … to other people." Their experiences were described as an "eye opener … you look at everything a little differently. … You can't judge people. … You never know what they've gone through." Parents described a "loss of innocence" and a "sense of powerlessness" over events in their lives at the same time they "gained an appreciation of life more … how fragile it is, and that it can go so easily. … You need to treasure it and take every moment."

When asked what advice they would have for other parents facing the loss of their infant, the most participants responded not to "take things for granted … just realize that there's no guarantees of anything … nothing at all," that people are "not immune from all the things you read." Not taking family and friends for granted became more important. "It makes you want to pick up the phone and just call and talk. … Let them know your feelings for them … you never know from 1 day to the next."

Parents also spoke of becoming stronger and better people for having lived through this terrible ordeal. One mother who was able to take her daughter home for a brief period affirmed that "part of the healing, I think, was how it changed me to be a better person. My life is very rich because of her … much more full and much more rich … and I see things in a totally different light, and I am so glad … that she came and that she went. … God really molded me into a totally different person because of her existence." One father felt that "it's obviously helped us to be more sensitive to people who have experienced the same thing. … I think it has helped us … well, I think we're stronger people. … You don't go through something like this and survive it … including our marriage … we've, we've figured out that we've been to the depths of hell, and we've survived … not only as individuals but as a couple, and I know a lot of times that doesn't happen." One mother felt that she "can't be worse because that's a very shameful legacy to leave my child … a mom that's worse because of her." Despite seeing themselves evolving into better people, all would "give it all up happily … to be selfish … to have him back." As one mother concluded, "It was rough, but we got through it, and we're better people for it …but I would rather have my daughter."

**SPIRITUAL/RELIGIOUS PERSPECTIVES**

Faith was a significant component for study participants as they went on with their daily lives. Some parents always were able to draw comfort from their faith: "That strong relationship I have with Him … I know carried me through that time," "Through the whole thing, I really felt very strongly that God just really gave me a strength I never knew I had; …you know that when they're with the Lord, there is nothing better." Others expressed anger at God while still embracing faith: "I am very angry at God, but I still attend church, I still talk to my priest. … I don't think I have anything else to hang onto but my faith." "I mean, I certainly went through a period where I was pretty mad … you know 'Why me? Why us? '… and I'm not ever going to have an answer to that, … but I guess the realization that He lost a son too … more than anything helped me to realize that He truly understands … all that we were going through." Still others abandoned the God of their childhood for belief in a higher being that is not all-powerful: "I had a hard time making sense of how this omniscient, omnipotent being could allow such horrible things to happen. … I was never able to reconcile my belief in God and what He does with the reality of life. … I think what I have now is a collection of what works for me, and I believe in a higher being, but I don't think he is all powerful because … children wouldn't die."

For many study participants it was the belief that their child was "in heaven, and we'll all be together one day" that "helps get me through." It was this "belief in an afterlife that makes it easier. I think if families don't have that, … that would be more difficult. I mean, if you really believe you die, and you go in the ground, and that's the end of you, that would be kind of scary and depressing."

Parents expressed a need for "something good to come out of something so bad." Viewing their child's death in a positive manner allowed parents to see the purpose in their infant's brief life and added to their spiritual foundation. As a father of an extremely premature infant described, "We tried to use this in a positive way in our lives, and … every night, as we get ready to go to sleep, we always have a prayer time together, and one of our prayers from the very beginning has always been, 'God, please use his life and allow us to be a part of it,' and that's still our prayer. We want good to come out of … what we had to go through, … and we want to be able to be a blessing to others, … to help others to walk through this thing." A mother of a daughter born with congenital anomalies felt that her daughter "also showed me a deeper compassion for those that are born with handicaps and disabilities, and what I have found myself doing after she passed away was just going out and trying to encourage other women who have lost children. … A year after she died I started a ministry in my church for parents who have lost children. … So that's one area, a huge area, where she really has changed my life. … And all this is a result of what she has meant and what she has done … done for me." Another mother came to the realization "that faith could keep growing, and I could keep learning more and more and more about faith and everything about God and everything how it affects our life and what we do, and I have to say, … it's intensified … that knowledge, that love, that foundation, … and I guess perspective on life, that that is what matters most … that is my … main goal … to teach that to my children … to show that to my children … to example that to my children, … because I just feel … one is delivered … to heaven."

## DISCUSSION

Deciding to withdraw life support from one's critically ill infant is a painful and overwhelming experience for parents. The participants' descriptions contained in this qualitative work provide an understanding of that decision as well their ongoing grief as they moved forward with their lives following the death of their infant. These rich descriptions entail movement over time as the parents incorporate not just memories but the continued essence of their deceased infant in their daily lives.

Consistently across the narratives was the parents' realization that further intervention on behalf of their infants was futile, and that there wasn't a "real choice" to be made other than to remove the infant from life support. Thus, believing that there was not a real decision to be made—that the infant was going to die with or without life support—study participants did not express regret or guilt over their decision but rather felt they did "the best they could under the circumstances." It was only in that time around removal of life support that parents spoke of regret in not having performed more parenting activities for their infant and in not having shared their infant more with others to provide them with additional cherished memories to be carried forward.

Because loss and grief are personal experiences, no specific formula for healing was identified. Parent participants uniformly stated that anyone in such a situation would need to determine what was and was not helpful for them personally and to listen to their hearts. Despite being able to move forward from the emotional turmoil incurred by the loss of their infant, all parents spoke of an ongoing void in their lives in the months and years following their infant's death that has become a part of their lives.

Parents found that their "whole view on life had changed" as they gained new perspectives that influenced how they conducted their lives and interacted with others as they went forward from their loss. Determined that their infant be more than remembered, it was imperative for parents to include their deceased infant as a part of their ongoing family structure. The deceased infant was not "left out" of family activities but maintained a rightful place in the evolving family structure.

Parents spoke of being better people because of their experience and because of the influence their infant continued to exert in their lives. The study participants wanted to be a live a life that would be worthy of the infant and to provide the infant with a proper "legacy." A belief in an afterlife provided them with the assurance that some day they would be re-united as a family.

This qualitative work provides unique insight into parents' perspectives of grief as they moved forward with their lives following the removal of life support and subsequent death of their infant. In addition it illuminates how parents' grief and loss becomes incorporated into their ongoing lives.

**REFERENCES**

1. Hoyert DL, Arias E, Smith BL, et al. Deaths: final data for 1999. Natl Vital Stat Rep 2001;49(8):11–3.
2. Wocial LD. Life support decisions involving imperiled infants. J Perinat Neonatal Nurs 2000;14(2):73–86.
3. Armentrout D. Holding a place: parents' lives following removal of infant life support. Newborn Infant Nurs Rev 2007;7(1):e3–8.
4. Armentrout D. Holding a place: a grounded theory of parents bringing their infant forward in their daily lives following the removal of life support and subsequent infant death [Doctoral dissertation, UMI No. 3167414]. Galveston (Texas): University of Texas Medical Branch; 2005.

# When the Fetus is Alive but the Mother is Not: Critical Care Somatic Support as an Accepted Model of Care in the Twenty-First Century?

Anita J. Catlin, DNSc, FNP, FAAN[a,*], Deborah Volat, BSN[b]

**KEYWORDS**

- Brain death • Pregnant • Somatic support
- Post-mortem cesarean section • Death with dignity

Advances in technology continue to create both opportunities and dilemmas in maternal/child nursing. The use of ventilator support, circulatory management, and artificial nutrition and hydration normally are used temporarily to allow a critically ill mother or infant to recover. The critical care nurse is able to manage artificially activities normally regulated by the healthy brain. If the brain does not recover and is deemed to be dead, technological therapeutics still can maintain the somatic activities. The debate as to whether any brain-dead person's body should be maintained to allow organ harvest has concluded in general acceptance of the practice, often allowing a few hours or days of life support while donation recipients are located. When tragedy strikes a pregnant woman, ending in her brain death, and she is used as a "harvest organ" for the developing fetus, the situation becomes more complex. This article describes the dilemma in which critical care and maternal/child nurses question whether a woman should be maintained on life support for periods up to 5 months or longer. Nurses are asking for guidance in understanding whether they should be providing life-extending therapeutics that may allow fetal development and birth from a mother who has died. Cases involving this ethical dilemma are increasing with increasing knowledge about how to maintain a body somatically after death.

[a] Department of Nursing, Sonoma State University, 1801 E. Cotati Avenue, Rohnert Park, CA 94928, USA
[b] Oncology, John Muir Medical Center, Walnut Creek, CA 94598, USA
* Corresponding author.
*E-mail address:* catlin@sonoma.edu (A.J. Catlin).

Crit Care Nurs Clin N Am 21 (2009) 267–276
doi:10.1016/j.ccell.2009.01.004 **ccnursing.theclinics.com**
0899-5885/09/$ – see front matter 

## TERMS

In this article, the following definitions are used:

Pregnant woman: a woman who is known or not known to be pregnant with a live fetus at the time of a life-limiting event

Brain-dead: the cessation of activity of the brain resulting from cerebral neurologic catastrophe as measured by (1) neuroimaging evidence, (2) exclusion of a confounding medical condition, (3) absence of drug intoxication, and (4) core temperature higher than 32°C and evidenced by coma, the absence of brainstem reflexes, and apnea[1]

Brain-dead pregnant woman (BDPW): a pregnant woman who has been determined to be brain dead. (Other terms used to describe the pregnant brain-dead woman in the literature include postmortem or perimortem pregnancy, cadaveric pregnancy, maternal organism, and posthumous motherhood. Although there is additional literature that describes the pregnant woman in a persistent vegetative state and the cognitively unaware pregnant woman, this article discusses only cases involving a BDPW. It has been estimated that 1060 pregnant women suffer brain death annually worldwide.)[2]

Somatic support: the physiologic support of the body to maintain heartbeat and respiration

## STATISTICS

Worldwide, there are approximately 22 published reports of BDPW who were maintained on technological life support to allow fetal development. These reports come from Brazil,[2] Germany,[3,4] Ireland,[5,6] New Zealand,[7] France,[8] Finland,[9] Korea,[10] Spain,[11] and the United States.[12–21] Causes of the brain death found in the literature included stroke, ruptured arterial-venous malformation, closed head injury, meningitis, intercranial mass lesion, melanoma, motor vehicle accident, firearm accident, and cocaine abuse. In all but two cases, the fetus was brought to a state of viability and lived after birth. In two cases,[3,11] the maternal pathophysiology was too extensive for the BDPW to be maintained on life support, and the fetus miscarried. Vives and colleagues[11] from Spain stated that they published their unsuccessful case study to counteract the many published reports that they believed were biased in favor of those fetuses that lived.

## DECISION MAKING

When a pregnant woman seems to be dying, every effort, of course, is made to save her life. The use of cardiopulmonary resuscitation, uterus emptying, and crash cesarean section as resuscitation has been discussed elsewhere.[22] When the woman cannot be saved and is deemed to be brain dead, Mallampalli and Guy[16] stated that one of three choices must be made: (1) to attempt to immediately deliver the fetus dependent upon the level of viability; (2) to continue full support of the woman's body to allow the fetus to mature; or (3) to discontinue mechanical support and allow the woman who has died to have technologies ended; the fetus will expire also.

The earliest gestational age at which fetal support in a BDPW was attempted was 13 weeks' gestation;[3] this fetus was miscarried shortly after support was attempted. Suddaby and colleagues[20] report a live birth with support beginning at 15 weeks' and continuing to 32 weeks' gestation. Others report extending somatic support for BDPW ranging from 16 to 36 weeks' gestation and achieving live birth outcomes. The longest sustained BDPW found in the literature occurred in 1989; Bernstein and colleagues[12] maintained this woman for 107 days after diagnosis of brain death at 15 weeks' gestation.

## MEDICAL AND NURSING CARE NEEDS

The care needed to support a BDPW somatically is similar to that needed for any person maintained on life support with the additional focus of ensuring adequate blood flow through the placenta. Before making a decision to continue the pregnancy, one would assess whether the fetus has a chance for healthy survival and whether additional family members desiring to raise the fetus/newborn exist. Feldman and colleagues[14] recommend ruling out any chromosomal abnormalities, neural tube defects, or congenital fetal anomalies.

This care would need to be undertaken in a hospital with high-level ICUs to sustain the woman and the neonate, if born, and well-trained antepartum, postpartum, and neonatal staff members. Somatic support of the woman would take place in an ICU with full capabilities for ventilation and resuscitation, access to an operating room, and a neonatal ICU. **Table 1** summarizes the somatic support necessary as delineated by Mallampalli and Guy,[16] Mallampalli, Powner, and Gardner,[17] and Powner and Bernstein.[18] In addition to physiologic support, Milliez and Cayol[8] discuss the need for dignity and compassion. **Table 2** describes ongoing support for the developing fetus.

## ETHICAL DELIBERATIONS

The ethical ramifications of this situation are vast. These questions relate to the woman, the fetus, the family, and the nursing staff. The ethical questions involve basic definitions of what is life and what is death and who is alive and who is dead. Ethical questions place Kant's admonition not to use a person as a means to an end against the dictum of Mill's utilitarianism dictum to maximize happiness for the most people.

### *Ethical Issues Related to the Mother*

Among the ethical questions related to the mother are

- Should the BDPW be treated with life-extending technology as if alive?
- Is it ethical to provide treatment to her body without consent?
- Does attending prenatal care visits constitute the acceptance of treatment on behalf of a fetus?
- If she had written an advance directive that asked for "no heroics," would this directive be overridden?
- Does filling out a card for organ donation constitute acceptance of life-extending therapies?
- Can keeping the fetus alive be likened to organ donation?
- Who is the appropriate surrogate decision maker for the BDPW?
- What if there is conflict about the decision?

Sperling,[23] in a 50-page legal and ethical brief, attempted to answer these questions. He reported complications, contradictions, and complexities in the ethics and the law. The authors suggest these questions be answered on a case-by-case basis, with inclusion of the hospital ethics committee.

**Table 1**
**Needs of the woman's body**

| | |
|---|---|
| Homeostasis | Intravenous fluids, crystalloids and colloids<br>Central lines<br>Maintenance of pH regulation |
| Blood pressure maintenance | Inotropics<br>Vasopressors with caution |
| Nutrition[a] | Nitrogen and fats by enteral or parental administration<br>Albumin<br>Vitamins, folic acid, and trace elements<br>Iron and iodine<br>Daily weights, for attempted weight gain of 25–35 pounds |
| Positioning and skin | Left lateral<br>Frequent turning and skin care<br>Special mattress<br>Heel and elbow protectors<br>Prophylactic heparin |
| Suppression of diabetes insipidus | Desmopressin<br>Salt regulation |
| Endocrine replacement | Thyroid hormone<br>Corticosteroids<br>Insulin for euglycemia |
| Respirations | Mechanical ventilation,<br>$PaCO_2$ 30–35<br>$PaO_2$ 105 |
| Temperature regulation | Warming blankets as needed for hypothermia<br>Prevention of hyperthermia |
| Infection protection | Antibiotics<br>Frequent cultures for gram-negative, gram-positive, and fungal pathogens<br>Strict infection control |
| Antibody suppression if Rh negative | Rhogam |
| Control of uterine contractions | Tocolytics |
| Organ donation | Contact with United Network for Organ Sharing and Transplantation (www.unos.com) if woman was designated donor or family wishes to donate other organs |
| Family issues | Weekly progress reports and family conferences. Pastoral care, social support, religious service (as culturally appropriate) at time of somatic support removal. |

[a] See Ref.[9] for a complete discussion.

### *Ethical Issues Related to the Fetus*

The status of the fetus also entails multiple ethical questions.

If the woman is dead, is her fetus alive?
Should the care providers be concerned with bringing the fetus to viability and birth as if it were an individual with the right to treatment?
Should weeks to months of extensive medical care and costs be devoted to obtain this individual life?

**Table 2**
**Needs of the fetus**

| | |
|---|---|
| Assessment of fetal development | Measurement of fetal heart rate<br>Non stress tests<br>Biophysical profile<br>Ultrasound measurements<br>Amniocentesis |
| Lung development | Betamethasone<br>Surfactant testing |
| Ability to deliver | Emergency cesarean section set-up |
| Time of delivery | Baptism or religious blessings at time of birth as desired by family |

Is this care an experimental treatment to which neither the woman nor the fetus can or has consented?

Does maintenance of life support on behalf of the fetus violate a woman's right to die with dignity?

The case studies from around the world tend to reflect the religious climate of the country in which the study was conducted. In an article from Ireland,[6] for example, the fetus's right to life is expressed. In a legal brief from New Zealand,[7] a more secular country, limitations on the legal rights of the fetus are defined. All authors seem to agree that this procedure would be considered experimental in nature.

### *Ethical Issues Related to the Family*

If no family steps forward, the woman probably would be allowed to die with dignity. If a family or loved ones do exist and are present in a timely manner, they will be asked their opinions on life-sustaining events. One hopes there will be no disagreements among family members reminiscent of the Terri Schiavo[24] case. (In the Schiavo case, the parents of Mrs. Schiavo wanted to continue her somatic support with artificial feeding while she was in a persistent vegetative state, and her husband wished to remove the feeding tube and allow her to die with dignity, as he stated was her expressed wish. This disagreement caused widespread judicial and ethical debate throughout the world.)

If the father of the fetus is identifiable and involved, he most likely would have input in the decision making. Hales[25] has written about such fathers' rights in pregnancy-related decision making. On the other hand, feminist scholars would want what is best for the woman and her interests. Purdy,[26] Sherwin,[27] and Lindemann[28] have written in opposition to using the woman as a "fetal container" and in support of her being allowed to die with dignity.

In the excitement over "saving" the fetus, questions must be answered to ascertain whether the family truly is prepared to care for an infant whose condition cannot be assured and who will not have a mother. Family counseling is needed, and there must be no shame for families who recognize that an already stressed grandmother or father with many other responsibilities may not be able to accept an additional burden, and that the living children may suffer neglect or other consequences by privileging the fetus.

### *Ethical Issues Related to the Nursing Staff*

Nurses and other members of the caregiving team may experience multiple and conflicting feelings. Although caring for the BDPW may seem altruistic and the ethical thing to do, in reality, caring for the brain-dead patient for extensive periods has not previously been done. A search of the Cumulative Index to Nursing and Allied Health Literature database revealed no nursing articles on caring for the BDPW and only two articles written in the past 10 years on caring for the brain-dead organ donor. Day[29] interviewed nine critical care nurses who maintained brain-dead organ donors. The nurses interviewed reported difficultly in changing from caring for a living patient to caring for a patient determined to be brain dead. This situation filled the nurses with ambiguity. The nurses turned their caring nursing activities to caring for the families while providing physiologic maintenance to the brain-dead patients. Sadala and Mendes[30] from Brazil asked 18 critical care nurses about their feelings when caring for brain-dead organ donors. These nurses referred to the donor as "a dead person, but a special dead person because the heart is beating." These authors also reported the nurses' feelings of ambiguity in caring for a patient "who is neither a person nor a thing" and in trying to identify the object of their nursing. In both studies nurses described the need to detach from thinking about the donor and to focus instead on the family and the potential donation. Sadala and Mendez[30] wrote that helping nurses believe that something positive comes out of the process is essential.

The feelings of nurses caring for a BDPW probably are similar to, or even more intense than, those described by Sadala and Mendez.[30] The extensive periods needed to bring the fetus to viability (as compared with the limited transience of brain death for organ donation) may cause nurses significant moral distress. Caring for the brain-dead physical body for long periods may be frightening or distasteful. Loczin,[31] a nursing expert who has written a text on the meaning of technology in nursing, has stated:

> *Technology and competence enhance effective caring, yet it is being observed that technology also impedes care by alienating and dehumanizing both the nurse and the patient, particularly when technological competence is not skillfully blended with sensitivity to the needs and responses of the patient.*

He continues:

> *Central to this … is the view that persons are not human bodies identified only as objects, but rather they are individuals who possess values of dignity and autonomy and who strive to live their hopes, dreams, and aspirations as persons.*

Locsin's text, published in 2005, does not address the influence of technology on care of the dead person who can no longer express his or her needs or hopes and dreams. Perhaps keeping the fetus alive is the family members' assumption of these dreams.

No position statement or guidance for nurses on the BDPW issue was found in a review of material from the Association of Women's Health, Obstetric and Neonatal Nursing, the American Operating Room Nurses, the American Association of Critical Care Nurses, or the National Association of Neonatal Nurses. The American Nurses Association had no position statement, but the Provision One of the Code of Ethics for Nurses[32] may give some assistance:

> *The nurse, in all professional relationships, practices with compassion and respect for the inherent dignity, worth, and uniqueness of every individual, unrestricted by considerations of social or economic status, personal attributes, or the nature of health problems.*

Thus the American Nurses Association would support the nurse who wished to consider the brain-dead person as a unique individual and worthy of nursing care.

Yet a nurse would have to agree voluntarily to provide this type of care for the BDPW. As Sadala and Mendes wrote, the nurse would have to find positive meaning in the actions. If nurse feels that providing this care would create a value conflict, and that keeping a body alive for the sake of another is not right, conscientious objection[33] would be appropriate.

## CARE IN THE ICU

If a BDPW is accepted in a critical care unit for somatic support, collaboration between the obstetric nurses and intensive care nurses will be ongoing. The obstetric nurses will come to the ICU daily (or more often) to do the non-stress testing, to palpate the abdomen for evidence of uterine rigidity or contractions, and to detect active fetal movement. The ICU nurses will be doing overall assessment and would note any perineal leaking, bleeding, or abnormal discharge. Fungal infections may occur, and rupture of membranes may manifest only as a slight but persistent leak of fluid. A change in the color of discharge to pink-tinged or an increased discharge of mucus may indicate cervical effacement and impending labor. Having the obstetric nurse there to evaluate and teach ICU nurses about subtle signs of change (such as sudden periodic spikes in maternal heart rate caused by contractions) enhances the ICU nurses' observation skills and care. The manner of delivery is a scheduled cesarean section when fetal lung maturity is established, but cervical dilation and vaginal delivery have occurred in a comatose, brain-injured woman being given somatic support for an extended period.[34]

As the fetus develops, three-dimensional color Doppler examinations are ongoing. Although the nurses may not bond to the BDPW, all concerned may develop an attachment to the fetus. As the day for delivery of the fetus approaches, new psychologic issues of separation and closure may arise, quite different from the experience ICU nurses have with the shorter-term stays of critically ill patients. These nurses will need leadership support, pastoral care, or psychiatry support services.

It is important to have a close working relationship between the intensive care and maternal/child nurses. Although the maternal/child team may be excited about participating in bringing the fetus to life, the intensive care nurses have provided long-term care for a brain-dead person who is decompensating. When the maternal/child team's job is about to begin, the intensive care nurses' job will come to an end. Weekly meetings that include both teams and that show respect for the difficult work of the ICU nurses are essential. All involved will experience a roller coaster of emotions.

Another group of nurses who may need support are the operating room nurses who care for the woman (and neonate) during and after the cesarean section. When and how the ventilator is removed has not been described in the literature. Shrader[19] has described the removal of life support from a BDPW as "dying more than one death." Nurses participating in these actions also need leadership support and critical incident debriefing. Future research will require both qualitative and quantitative assessment and analyses of both nurses' and physicians' experiences surrounding this still rare, but growing, phenomenon. A memorial service for the mother might help all staff process what they have experienced.

## FINANCIAL ISSUES

The cost of maintaining a brain-dead person on life support depends on the number of days spent in the ICU. One might consider that every day (after viability) that the fetus is in utero is a day in which fetal development occurs and represents 1 day less that the fetus would have to be in the neonatal ICU. Those concerned with social justice and health care for all children might question this type of financial effort on behalf of one child. It is uncertain if government or private insurance would pay for this type of extended care. The cost–benefit analysis of maintaining somatic functioning in a brain-dead woman is increasingly weighed against the overall unavailability of ICU beds, the scarcity of other resources and nursing staff, and limited access to health care in general.

## RECOMMENDATIONS

The ethical debate over BDPW seems to the authors to be one of a personal nature. One must decide on two issues: (1) is there is a inherent wrongness in using a BDPW as an incubator for the fetus; and (2) is the fetus healthy enough and gestationally mature enough that trying to save it will not be distasteful to the care providers? Classical ethical principles do not seem to work: neither the woman nor the fetus has autonomy, neither can give informed consent, and neither can refuse treatment. Some may find beneficence (doing the good thing) in trying to save a fetus; others may state that this attempt is the most maleficent (doing harm as a result of trying to do good) and worst thing they have ever heard of. It seems that if a family wishes to take this course, if the fetus is healthy, if the facility is willing to absorb the cost for the long-term care, and if there are physicians and nurses who wish to participate, then the attempt might be made. Any person who finds this attempt distasteful would have the option of not serving on the team.

It also seems that more guidance from pregnant women is needed. The movement to increase the use of the advance directive is widespread, encouraged mostly for older adults who have chronic conditions to make their wishes known should they become incapacitated. The Five Wishes document is an outstanding version of the Advance Directive.[35] Catlin[36] has suggested that this document be extended for a pregnant woman to state her desires in advance on how she wishes fetal emergencies, such as extremely premature labor, to be handled. In her work, Catlin refers only to directives for what the healthy woman would want should the fetus or newborn have a life-limiting condition. Neither form of directive mentions a pregnant woman's directives for her fetus should she die during the pregnancy. No legal document has asked the pregnant woman what she would want done with her fetus upon her incapacitation. Now that the technology for somatic support exists, it is essential to add this feature to the advance directive of any woman of childbearing age and perhaps to include it in the standard prenatal interview.

Thirty-five years ago, Willard Gaylin,[37] the co-founder of the Hastings Ethics Center, predicted that this type of technological maintenance of somatic functioning would occur. He wrote a fascinating science fiction–type scenario describing the brain-dead cadaver being kept alive as a source of transplant organs and biologic resources, but even he did not predict the gestation of a fetus in a brain-dead mother. Now nurses are being asked to care in ways not envisaged in their training. A nurse must make an individual decision that best fits his or her values, share these values in a professional manner, and then walk forward into the twenty-first century.

## ACKNOWLEDGMENTS

The authors thank Dr. Laura Malmeister, historian Lauren Coodley, MA, and maternal child and perioperative director, Nance Jones, MSN, for their wisdom and excellent suggestions to the manuscript.

**REFERENCES**


1. American Academy of Neurology. Practice parameters for determining brain death in adults. The quality standards subcommittee of the American Academy of Neurology. Neurology 1995;45(5):1012–4.
2. Souza JP, Olivera-Neto A, Surita FG, et al. The prolongation of somatic support in a pregnant woman with brain-death: a case report. Reprod Health 2006;3:3.
3. Anstotz C. Should a brain-dead pregnant woman carry her child to full term? The case of the "Erlanger baby". Bioethics 1993;7(4):340–50.
4. Wuermeling HB. Brain-death and pregnancy. Forensic Sci Int 1994;69(3):243–5.
5. Farragher R, Marsh B, Laffey IG. Maternal brain death—an Irish perspective. Ir J Med Sci 2005;174(4):55–9.
6. Lane A, Westbrook A, Grady D, et al. Maternal brain death: medical, ethical and legal issues. Intensive Care Med 2004;30:1484–6.
7. Peart NS, Campbell AV, Manara AR, et al. Maintaining pregnancy following loss of capacity. Med Law Rev 2000;8:275–99.
8. Milliez J, Cayol V. Palliative care with pregnant women. Best Pract Res Clin Obstet Gynaecol 2001;15(2):323–31.
9. Nuutinen LS, Alahuhta SM, Heikkinen JE. Nutrition during ten-week life support with successful fetal outcome in a case with fatal maternal brain damage. JPEN J Parenter Enteral Nutr 1989;13(4):432–5.
10. Sim KB. Maternal persistent vegetative state with successful fetal outcome. J Korean Med Sci 2001;16:669–72.
11. Vives A, Carmona F, Zabala E, et al. Maternal brain death during pregnancy. Int J Gynaecol Obstet 1996;52:67–9.
12. Bernstein IM, Watson M, Simmons GM, et al. Maternal brain death and prolonged fetal survival. Obstet Gynecol 1989;74(3, Part 2):S437–9.
13. Bush M, Nagy S, Berkowitz RL, et al. Pregnancy in a persistent vegetative state: case report, comparison to brain death, and review of the literature. Obstet Gynecol Surv 2003;58(11):738–48.
14. Feldman DM, Borgida AF, Rodis JF, et al. Irreversible maternal brain injury during pregnancy: a case report and review of the literature. Obstet Gynecol Surv 2000; 55(11):708–14.
15. Lewis DD, Vidovich RR. Organ recovery following childbirth by a brain-dead mother: a case report. J Transpl Coord 1997;7(3):103–5.
16. Mallampalli A, Guy E. Cardiac arrest in pregnancy and somatic support after brain death. Crit Care Med 2005;33(10):S325–31.
17. Mallampalli A, Powner DJ, Gardner M. Cardiopulmonary resuscitation and somatic support of the pregnant patient. Crit Care Clin 2004;20:747–61.
18. Powner DJ, Bernstein IM. Extended somatic support for pregnant women after brain death. Crit Care Med 2003;31(4):1241–9.
19. Shrader D. On dying more than one death. February. Hastings Cent Rep 1986; February:12–7.
20. Suddaby EC, Schaeffer MJ, Brigham LE, et al. Analysis of organ donors in the peripartum period. J Transpl Coord 1999;8(1):35–9.
21. Yeung P Jr, Mcmanus C, Tchabo JG. Extended somatic support for a pregnant woman with brain death from metastatic malignant melanoma: a case report. J Matern Fetal Neonatal Med 2008;21(7):509–11.
22. Katz V, Balderston K, Defreest M. Perimortem cesarean delivery: were our assumptions correct. Am J Obstet Gynecol 2005;192:1916–21.
23. Sperling D. Maternal brain death. Am J Law Med 2004;30:453–500.

24. Caplan AL, McCartney JJ, Sisti DA, editors. The case of Terri Schiavo: ethics at the end of life. Amherst (NY): Prometheus Books; 2006.
25. Hales S. In: Humber JM, Almeder RF, editors. Reproduction, technology, and rights. New Jersey: Human Press; 1996.
26. Purdy LM. Are pregnant women fetal containers? Bioethics 2007;4(4):273–91.
27. Sherwin S. No longer patient: feminist ethics and health care. Philadelphia: Temple University Press; 1992.
28. Lindemann-Nelson H. The architect and the bee: reflections on postmortem pregnancy. Bioethics 1994;8(3):247–67.
29. Day LJ. How nurses shift from care of a brain-injured patient to maintenance of a brain-dead organ donor. Am J Crit Care 2001;10(5):306–12.
30. Sadala MLA, Mendes HWB. Caring for organ donors: the intensive care unit nurses' view. Qual Health Res 2000;10(6):788–805.
31. Loczin RC. Technological competency as caring in nursing. Indianapolis (IN): Sigma Theta Tau; 2005.
32. Fowler MDM, editor. Guide to the code of ethics for nurses. Silver Springs (MD): American Nurses Association; 2008.
33. Catlin AJ, Armigo C, Volat D, et al. Conscientious objection: a possible nursing response to care at the end of life which is harmful, causes suffering, or torture. Neonatal Netw 2008;27(2):101–6, 107–8.
34. Sampson MB, Petersen LP. Post-traumatic coma during pregnancy. Obstet Gynecol 1979;53(3 Suppl):2S–3S.
35. Aging with Dignity. Five wishes document. Available at: http://www.agingwithdignity.org/5wishes.html. Accessed August 11, 2008.
36. Catlin A. Thinking outside the box: prenatal care and the call for a prenatal advance directive. J Perinat Neonatal Nurs 2005;19(2):169–76.
37. Gaylin W. Harvesting the dead. Harpers 1974;249(1492):23–30.

# When Neonatal ICU Infants Participate in Research: Special Protections for Special Subjects

Karen A. Thomas, PhD

**KEYWORDS**

- Research ethics • Neonatal intensive care
- Neonate • Premature infant • Parental consent
- Government regulation

Advances in neonatal ICU (NICU) practices are based on research findings from studies conducted among high-risk infants. With the continuing emphasis on evidence-based practice, there is an ongoing need for research in this vulnerable population, but special federal restrictions apply to research involving children. Understanding the regulations governing research among NICU patients is important in both neonatal nursing research and practice. Researchers must be cognizant of federal requirements pertaining to research with children and apply this information in the design and conduct of research. In the practice setting, neonatal nurses may conduct clinical research projects and implement research protocols. Nurses play important roles in protecting patients' safety, including safe participation in research.[1] Nurses' commitment to ethical practice includes protecting the rights of infants who participate in research.[2] Further, nurses serve as resources for parents who consent to their infant's participation in research. This article describes the federal regulations pertaining to the definition of neonates as a vulnerable population, the determination of risk in neonatal research, and the need for parental consent.

The protection of human research subjects is governed by the Code of Federal Regulations Title 45, Public Welfare, Department of Health and Human Services, Part 46 (45CFR46).[3] These federal policies apply to all research conducted by any agency that is subject to federal regulation. Most commonly, compliance with these regulations is connected with receipt of federal money, such as grants and contracts, and involves agencies funded directly by the federal government or those receiving

Department of Family and Child Nursing, University of Washington, 1959 NE Pacific Street, Seattle, WA 98195, USA
*E-mail address:* kthomas@u.washington.edu

Crit Care Nurs Clin N Am 21 (2009) 277–281
doi:10.1016/j.ccell.2009.01.007 ccnursing.theclinics.com

federal dollars such as Medicare/Medicaid. Almost all health care facilities and universities fall under these regulations.

45CFR46 requires the review and approval of human research by an institutional review board (IRB). Generally hospitals, universities, health departments, and similar agencies manage IRBs internally; however, review of research involving human subjects also may be conducted by independent approved IRBs, and this form of review by an external IRB may involve the payment of fees. Members of an IRB include scientists with research experience and community members who review research protocols guided by the rules specified in 45CFR46 and the accepted ethical procedures for the conduct of research. Three main ethical principles guide the review of research: autonomy, beneficence, and justice. Autonomy or respect for persons refers to individuals' independent and voluntary participation in research and the protection of persons with diminished capacity. In essence the principle of beneficence means that the research must "do good." The benefits of the research must outweigh the risks involved in participation. Justice represents fair treatment and equitable distribution of the burden of research and the benefits across the population. Key elements of IRB review include determination of risks and benefits, minimization of risk, avoidance of coercive recruitment, and informed consent. The IRB critically examines the proposed research study in relation to federal requirements. The rules set forth in 45CFR46 are stated in broad terms, and IRB reviewers apply interpretations of the federal regulations. These interpretations may vary based on the experiences of the IRB as a whole, the composition of the IRB, and members' individual perspectives.

## NEONATES AS A PROTECTED GROUP

Children, including neonates, are defined by 45CFR46 as one of several vulnerable groups requiring extra protection in the conduct of research. (Other vulnerable groups are prisoners, individuals with diminished capacity, pregnant women when pregnancy is the basis for study inclusion, and fetuses.) The regulations pertaining to neonates of uncertain viability and nonviable neonates are particularly relevant in neonatal nursing research and practice. Inclusion of nonviable infants or infants of questionable viability in research requires all of the following:

1. There is scientific evidence of potential risks.
2. Parents or legal guardians are fully informed of the consequences of the research for the neonate.
3. Investigators have no role in determining viability of the neonate.
4. The research risk is completely caused by a procedure or intervention that holds the promise of direct benefit, or, if there is no direct benefit, the risk to the neonate is minimal.

Viable neonates fall under federal regulations for children's participation in research. The regulations provide for approval of research involving children under four categories that are differentiated by risk and possible direct benefit to the child. These regulations, as they apply to neonates, are summarized in **Table 1**. Although not discussed here, the child's assent in addition to parental consent must be considered for older children. In general, research involving more than minimal risk must provide direct benefit to the child or produce generalizable findings that will inform improvements for the care of those with the same disease or condition. The degree of risk is central to determining the type of children's research that may be approved by the IRB and involves defining minimal risk, discussed in the next section.

**Table 1**
**Categories of research that may be approved for neonates' participation**

| Regulation | Description of Research | Conditions | Parental Consent (46.408) |
|---|---|---|---|
| 46.404 | Research does not involve more than minimal risk | — | Single parent may provide consent |
| 46.405 | Research involving more than minimal risk but offering the promise of direct benefit to the individual infant subject | Benefits outweigh the risks, and the benefits are at least as favorable as available alternative approaches. | Single parent may provide consent |
| 46.406 | Research involving more than minimal risk and no direct benefit to the child but likely to produce generalizable findings about the child's disorder or condition | Risk is a minor increase over minimal, interventions and procedures are consistent with actual or expected medical, psychological, or social situations, the knowledge gained is vital to understanding or treating the infant's condition | Both parents must consent unless one parent is deceased, unknown, incompetent, or not reasonably available, or one parent has sole custody |
| 46.407 | Research not otherwise approvable (above) that provides an opportunity to understand, prevent, or alleviate a serious health problem affecting the health or welfare of infants | The research is likely to increase understanding, prevention, and alleviation of a serious health problem affecting the health or welfare of infants, and permission is granted by the Department of Health and Human Services following review by expert panel and opportunity for public review and comment | Both parents must consent unless one parent is deceased, unknown, incompetent, or not reasonably available, or one parent has sole custody. |

*Adapted from* Department of Health & Human Services. 45CFR46, D. Additional Protections for Children Involved as Subjects in Research. Code of Federal Regulations Title 45 Public Welfare Department of Health and Human Services Part 46 Protection of Human Subjects. 2005. Available at: http://www.hhs/gov/ohrp/humansubjects/guidance/45cfr46.htm.

## RESEARCH RISK DEFINED FOR NEONATES

Risk in research refers to the possibility of injury or harm. Minimal risk is defined in 45CFR46 as "the probability and magnitude of harm or discomfort anticipated in the research are not greater in and of themselves than those ordinarily encountered in daily life or during the performance of routine physical or psychological examinations or tests" (46.102(i)). The continuum of risk is not categorized easily into discrete categories such as minimal versus greater than minimal risk. Further, there are no specific federal definitions of risk in children. IRB members often hold differing views about what constitutes risk for subjects in general and for neonates in particular. Ambiguity in the regulatory language results in inconsistencies in IRB interpretation of regulations in reviewing research involving children.[4] IRBs are challenged to define harm or discomfort for a neonate, particularly neonates receiving intensive care. The probability and magnitude of harm also are important aspects in defining risk. How likely is the harm or injury, and how serious is the harm? A third consideration is comparison of risk to that experienced in typical daily activities or routine health care. Although not universally held, the use of a uniform standard comparing risk to that experienced by healthy children is recommended.[4] Routine health care associated with a well-child visit is proposed as a criterion for typical experiences. This recommendation suggests that normally developing, healthy, nonhospitalized neonates of similar age should be the basis for comparison when evaluating risk in research involving neonates. Preterm infants in the NICU, however, do not have nonhospitalized counterparts, and even elements of normal well-child visits, such as handling or a heel stick, may produce distress. When making comparisons with the experiences of healthy, normal neonates, the developmental limitations and health status of preterm infants are important considerations. Guidelines for examining risk for children include the duration and frequency of procedures, the total or cumulative risk involved in a series of procedures, and the transient and reversible nature of the harm produced.[4] For example, the risk related to a neonatal research protocol that involves a single, brief episode of handling would be evaluated differently from a protocol involving multiple and/or prolonged handling. The IRB's determination of minimal risk relies on pain or discomfort not being severe, the harm being transient and reversible, the investigators being skilled in the procedure, and the setting being appropriate.[4]

## PARENTAL CONSENT

As with all research involving children, consent for research participation is obtained from parents or legal guardians who act on behalf of the neonate. The term "parent" here refers to biologic parent or legal adoptive parent. Parents of NICU patients may be particularly challenged because of their desire to assure the best care for their infants and a willingness to take risks in the hope of improved outcome. In one study, parents of NICU patients were more likely to consent to research that involved moderate risk and possible major direct benefit than were parents of normal, healthy newborns.[5] When confronted with a request for participation in medical research, 81% of parents of NICU patients report trusting doctors to not do research that would put the baby in danger.[5] Parents may not fully appreciate risk and benefit. The same study found that nearly one third of the parents of NICU patients and of normal newborn infants would consent to a study with no direct benefit and moderate risk.[5] Parental consent for participation in research often is sought during a traumatic period when parents are distressed by the neonate's health and the parents themselves are vulnerable.[6] Guidelines for obtaining informed consent have been published.[7]

**Box 1**
**Web resources**

Office for Human Research Protections (OHRP), OHRP Research Involving Children Frequently Asked Questions. Available at: http://www.hhs.gov/ohrp/researchfaq.html.

Office for Human Research Protections (OHRP), Special Protections for Children as Research Subjects. Available at: http://hhs.gov/ohrp/children.

Federal regulations specify not only that informed parental consent be obtained but also whether one or both parents must provide consent based on the four categories of IRB-approvable research (**Table 1**). Consent from both parents is required when minimal risk is exceeded and the research does not provide direct benefit. When both parents' consent is needed, the biologic father must be included in the consent process unless the exceptions, listed in **Table 1**, apply. Paternity therefore is an issue related to parental consent.

## SUMMARY

Neonatal nurses, although providing direct care to neonates and their families, frequently are not consulted regarding participation in research. Although they perceive themselves as advocates for the best interests their clients, only 54% of neonatal nurses report being included in decision making regarding neonates' participation in research.[8] Federal regulations provide special protections for children, including neonates, who are involved in research. Nurses' knowledge of these regulations guides the conduct of clinical research and provides the basis for assuring protection of parents' and neonates' rights. **Box 1** lists resources that can provide further information about the protections safeguarding children who participate in research.

## REFERENCES


1. Thomas KA. Safety: when infants and parents are research subjects. J Perinat Neonatal Nurs 2005;19(1):52–8.
2. Franck LS. Research with newborn participants: doing the right research and doing it right. J Perinat Neonatal Nurs 2005;19(2):177–86.
3. Department of Health & Human Services. Code of federal regulations title 45 public welfare Department of health and human services part 46 protection of human subjects. 2005. Available at: http://www.hhs/gov/ohrp/humansubjects/guidance/45cfr46.htm. Accessed February 6, 2009.
4. Fisher CB, Kornetsky SZ, Prentice ED. Determining risk in pediatric research with no prospect of direct benefit: time for a national consensus on the interpretation of federal regulations. Am J Bioeth 2007;7(3):5–10.
5. Singhal N, Oberle K, Burgess E, et al. Parents' perceptions of research with newborns. J Perinatol 2002;22(1):57–63.
6. McKechnie L, Gill AB. Consent for neonatal research. Arch Dis Child Fetal Neonatal Ed 2006;91(5):F374–76.
7. Golec L, Gibbins S, Dunn MS, et al. Informed consent in the NICU setting: an ethically optimal model for research solicitation. J Perinatol 2004;24(12):783–91.
8. Monterosso L, Kristjanson L, Sly PD, et al. The role of the neonatal intensive care nurse in decision-making: advocacy, involvement in ethical decisions and communication. Int J Nurs Pract 2005;11(3):108–17.

# Index

*Note:* Page numbers of article titles are in **boldface** type.




Crit Care Nurs Clin N Am 21 (2009) 283–291
doi:10.1016/S0899-5885(09)00032-X
ccnursing.theclinics.com

## G



## H



## I



## L

**R**

## S

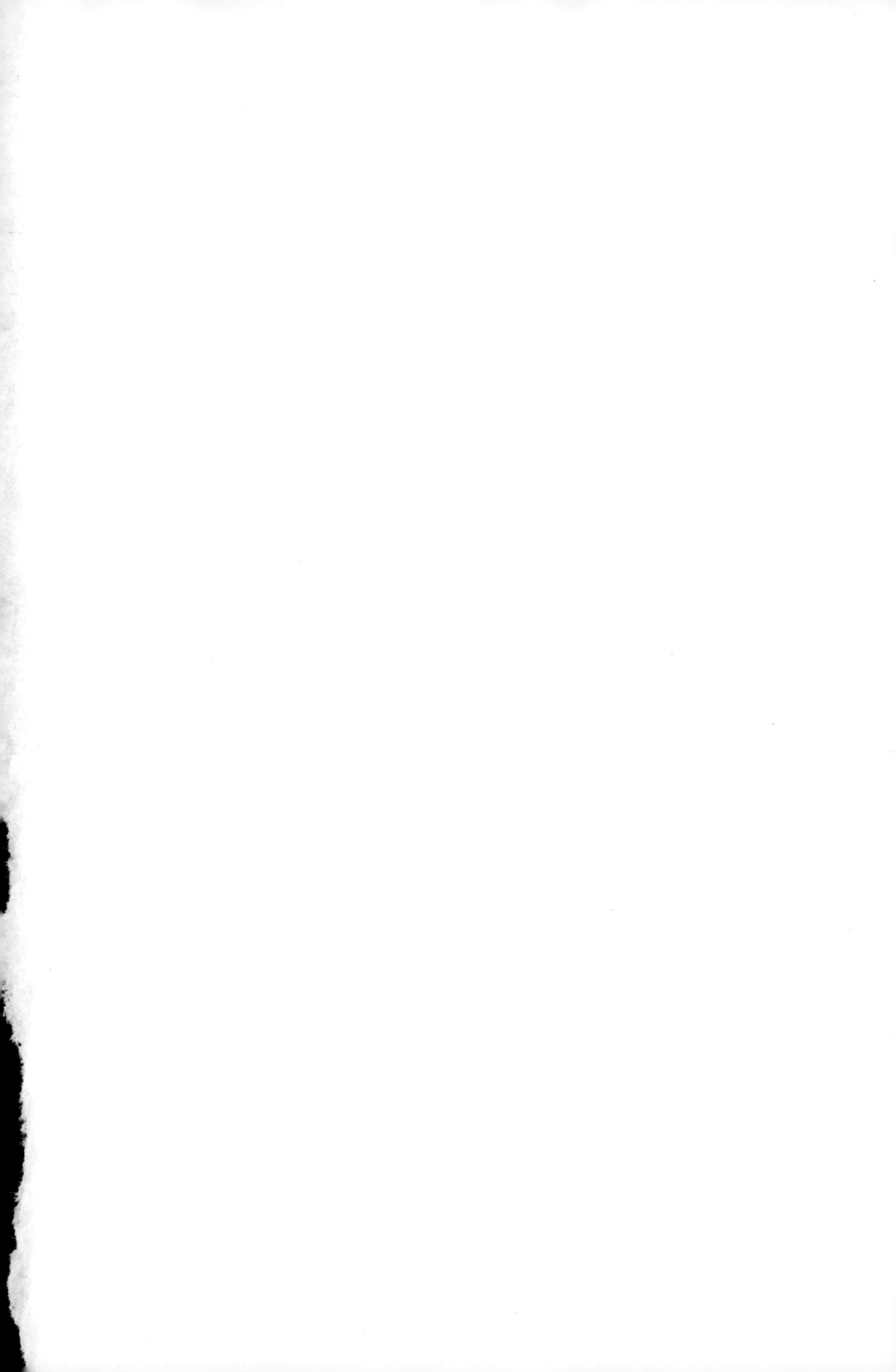

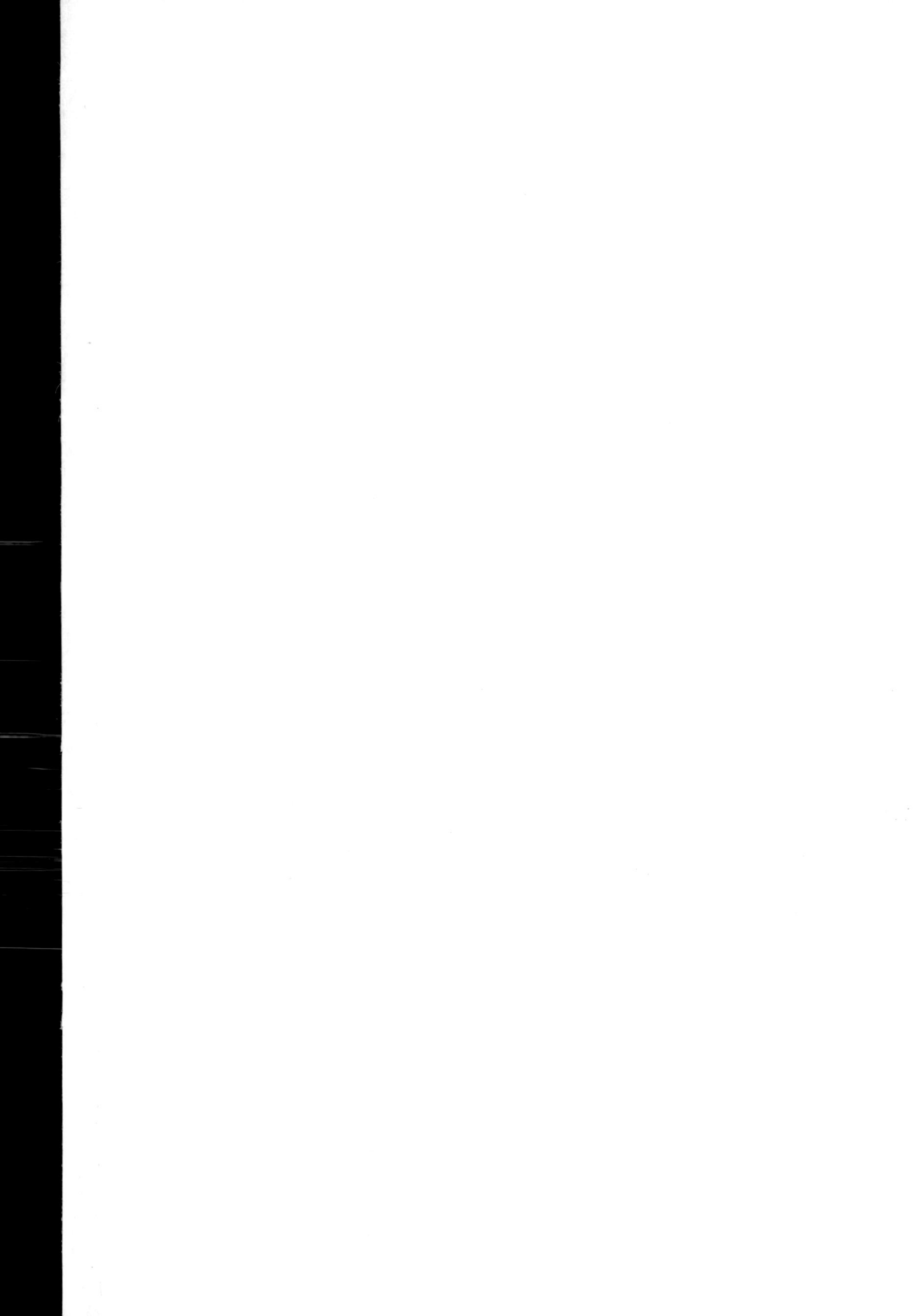